The Philosophy of Public Health

Benjamin Smart

The Philosophy of Public Health

A Capacities Approach

palgrave
macmillan

Benjamin Smart
B-Ring 703, The Centre for Philosophy
of Epidemiology, Medicine and Public Health
University of Johannesburg
Johannesburg, South Africa

ISBN 978-3-031-98803-5   ISBN 978-3-031-98804-2 (eBook)
https://doi.org/10.1007/978-3-031-98804-2

This Palgrave Macmillan imprint is published by the registered company Springer Nature Switzerland AG.
The registered company address is: Gewerbestrasse 11, 6330 Cham, Switzerland

To the memory of South Africa's late, great, selfless freedom fighters. To Nelson Mandela, Oliver Tambo, Steve Biko, Chris Hani, Walter and Albertina Sisulu, Pravin Gordhan (whom I had the pleasure of meeting), Tito Mboweni (whose recipes I avoided like the plague), and countless others—many of whom I will likely never know about. Their contribution to the health of South Africa's population (as health is understood in this book) must never be forgotten.

Introduction

In February 2020, the video footage from hospitals in Italy started filtering through into our living rooms. The hospitals were beyond full capacity. Hundreds of people unable to breathe. Dying. It was like something out of a horror movie. Shortly afterwards, we received news that the first case of COVID-19 had been recorded in South Africa. The tension rose, and the South African Government set up The National Coronavirus Command Council, which comprised mainly NatJoints (the country's national security committee), along with some eminent figures in epidemiology and public health. What followed, motivated the writing of this book.

In March 2020, the citizens of South Africa were informed that government would be "following the science", whatever that was supposed to mean. It turned out that following the science meant locking the whole country (minus those working in essential services) inside their homes, except to receive medical attention or to buy groceries. At first for three weeks, but lockdown persisted in various (progressively relaxed) forms for over a year. The sale of cigarettes was banned (with no evidence that this was an effective preventative measure), taking away a psychological crutch for many South Africans and sparking a surge in the illicit cigarette market. The same for alcohol. The sale of all kinds of goods was banned, including, somewhat bizarrely, open-toed shoes and children's toys. After a few months, citizens were briefly allowed to leave their homes for exercise early in the morning. For some reason, government demanded citizens all exercised at the same time, raising the probability of close contact with neighbours.

South Africa is the most unequal country in the world. The minority live in nice middle-class houses, often in security estates. They typically have a regular income, their children go to the kinds of school able to provide online learning, and they could work from home and maintain their income. The majority live in relative (or actual) poverty. They live in high-population density townships, informal settlements constructed from corrugated iron, and dilapidated urban areas. They mostly work in the informal sector, live hand-to-mouth, and the schools their children attend typically do not have the resources to provide online learning. For the majority, lockdown meant a choice between compliance and food insecurity/possible starvation, and non-compliance. Unsurprisingly, many chose non-compliance. The non-compliance led to a surge in police brutality, with the Institute for Security Services reporting: "Numerous videos on social media [showing] police and soldiers kicking, slapping and whipping alleged transgressors and forcing them to perform demeaning actions whilst laughing and making fun of them" (ISS 2020).

Lockdown in South Africa severely affected the economy, resulting in the loss of 671,000 jobs in the first quarter of 2020, in a country which already has the highest unemployment rate in the world. Government set aside an emergency budget of ZAR500 billion (around US $25 billion), much of which would later disappear into the pockets of corrupt opportunistic tenderpreneurs. The effect on other healthcare services was devastating. HIV testing programmes were stopped, non-essential surgeries were stopped, and vaccination programmes were slowed. Many people lost their lives through an inability to access medical services. This number included a friend of ours, who passed away after showing up to a government hospital with severe jaundice, but was never seen to. He'd waited the whole day without seeing a medical professional, and decided the risk of getting COVID-19 wasn't worth the benefit of waiting any longer.

When the vaccines arrived, there was a very mixed reaction. Many were very keen to protect themselves, but many others were hesitant. I was interviewed on the national news and asked whether I thought the vaccines would somehow interact with 5G technology, and whether Bill Gates would be tracking our every movement via computer chips. It's extraordinary what some will believe in the right circumstances. Uptake was relatively poor, but given the risk factors of COVID-19, and the relatively young average age of South Africans (compared to, e.g., Italians), the death toll was ultimately far lower than projected. At the time of writing, nearly five years after the outbreak of COVID-19 in South Africa, a little over 100,000 are confirmed to have died from the disease. That is a lot of people, but context is important. South Africa loses roughly 60,000 people to tuberculosis every year.

The COVID-19 era was a time of great stress, and for many, a time of loss. The public health decisions made by government affected so many people. There are, no doubt, many people alive in South Africa today, who would not be had government not locked the country down in early 2020. Nonetheless, the logic of many of their decisions remains lost on me.

In this book, I consider what it means to "follow the science" in situations akin to the COVID-19 pandemic. I look at what population health *is*, what the goals of public health are, and why it is important to strictly adhere to some of the basic tenets of evidence-based public health, even when there is great pressure (and need) to act, and act fast. I also consider some ontological questions pertaining to public health, and conclude the book with three chapters specifically focused on the ethics of public health. I develop a general ethical framework for public health (broadly construed) decision-making, consider what it might mean to decolonize public health, and whether decolonization should be pursued. Throughout, I argue that focusing on developing the capacities of both individuals and those of populations/societies as complex systems is key.

I have written this book from the perspective of a Western-trained, British philosopher, who has lived and worked in sub-Saharan Africa for a decade. Its insights are deeply affected by my experiences in South Africa, and many of the examples used in the book will be drawn from this context. I do not intend to "pick on" the South African government or its public health institutions. I do not question their intentions, nor the expertise of the country's public health specialists. No doubt, had I spent the pandemic in some other country, this book would be littered with similar examples from a different region. Generally speaking, this is not a book about philosophy of public health *in South Africa*. The account of population health I provide, the goals of public health I suggest, and the ontological and ethical conclusions are just as applicable in other contexts. They are, it is worth noting, prescriptive accounts. I am not describing the way health is currently understood, or how ethical dilemmas are currently approached. I am suggesting a new way of understanding health and the effects of this new approach on the goals of public health, the metaphysics of public health, health ethics, and decolonizing public health.

Approach

Entire books could be (and in some cases have been) written on the ethics of public health, on the metaphysics of public health, and indeed on the concept of health in public health. I nonetheless hope that I provide a convincing case for adopting the capacities approach to health, and that this work inspires others to note both their objections to my general approach (I would hope not too many of these focus on "this is not what public health does", since that would be to misunderstand the book's prescriptive intentions), develop the view, and hopefully find effective ways to apply the strategy in specific contexts.

Reference

ISS. 2020. Institute for Security Services. https://issafrica.org/iss-today/police-abuses-during-lockdown-reflect-deep-accountability-problems. Accessed 12 Nov 2024.

Acknowledgements

I would like to thank my wonderful wife, Emma, for her tireless love and support—you are a force of nature and the best thing that ever happened to me; our children, Mikey and Mila, for their effortless ability to make me smile; my parents, without whom I'd still be making rich people richer for a living; and my parents-in-law, Mike and Sue, for always being so welcoming and for being such wonderful grandparents.

I'd also like to thank my colleagues and co-authors for their support and/or useful feedback on earlier versions of the manuscript and related talks. Notably: Alex Broadbent, Hennie Lotter, Sridhar Venkatapuram, Michael Talibard, Elodie Giroux, Somogy Varga, Thaddeus Metz, Herculaas Combrink, Daniel Novotny, Dimpho Takane-Maponya, Chris Wareham, Chadwin Harris, Veli Mitova, and our Executive Dean, Kammila Naidoo.

Contents

List of Figures

List of Tables

1

Healthy Parts, Healthy Organisms, and Healthy Populations

1.1 Outline

The first two chapters of this book address two fundamental (and related) questions in the Philosophy of Public Health: first, the nature of "health" when applied at the population level, and second, the goals of public health as a discipline/profession. Since public health (the discipline) can broadly be understood as having the "primary purpose of protecting and improving the health of the public" (Childress et al. 2002), before identifying the goals of public health, one must first understand what improving the health of the public amounts to. In this first chapter, I consider the view that "health" is a property at best applicable only metaphorically to populations, since a non-metaphorical reading would require reifying populations as if they were "a natural thing—an organic whole with its own interests, needs, and being" (Jennings 2007, p. 54) (See Giroux (2021) for further discussion). If populations are not "natural things", they argue, health can only truly be considered a property of individual organisms and their physiological parts. I reject this view, arguing instead that health is a property of complex biological systems, and further that

B. Smart, *The Philosophy of Public Health*,
https://doi.org/10.1007/978-3-031-98804-2_1

many animal populations, including some human populations, qualify as complex systems suitable for instantiating the health property.

Although there is relatively little work on the health property applied to populations, the philosophy of medicine literature is rife with attempts at analyzing health and disease at the level of the organism. This is typically presented as an exercise in conceptual analysis, but as Harriet Fagerberg (2023) and Mael Lemoine (2013) have recently pointed out, the authors rarely stick to the rules of engagement of genuine conceptual analysis. Counterexamples of conditions currently classified as diseases (but that do not come out as diseases under their analysis) are deemed not to be diseases, counterexamples of conditions not considered diseases by mainstream medicine (but come out as diseases under the author's analysis) are deemed to be diseases, and little attention is paid to the actual use of the terms, or the time and context-dependent nature of these concepts. Instead, as Fagerberg argues, these authors seem to be engaging more in the project of identifying the nature of diseases as real kinds; that is, picking out the cluster of properties that unify those conditions falling under the real kind "disease".

In this chapter, via analyses of disease, I focus on health. Mine is a prescriptive account, so I do not claim that the account of health provided is how the concept is currently understood; rather, it is an account that could usefully be employed by public health policymakers. The account I provide is applicable not only at the population level, but at all levels of biological complexity—the cell, the organ, the organism, and the population.

I acknowledge that concepts of health and disease are thoroughly context dependent. Its content may differ depending on needs, goals, and even cultural context. I have argued elsewhere (2016) that the "theoretical" concept of disease (Boorse 1977), for example, might differ substantially from the concept employed by physicians in the clinic. A value-free concept is plausible in the former case, but not in the latter, since clinicians must be concerned with the values of their patients.

Here, I argue that health, at all levels of complexity, is best understood as an emergent property of complex systems. Health is not, on my view, a mind-independent natural property. Nor is the content of the concept immune to changes over time. Following Lennart Nordenfelt (2018) (with respect to health at the organism-level), I suggest that the content of the health-concept at all levels of biological complexity should be guided by the value-laden "vital goals" of individuals (see Sect. 3).

Perhaps the most widely discussed analysis of disease is Christopher Boorse's Biostatistical Theory (BST). BST takes a purely reductive approach to health, defining it as "…the readiness of each internal part to perform all its normal functions on typical occasions with at least typical efficiency." (Boorse 2014). An organism is thus unhealthy (diseased) should at least one of their internal parts fail to perform with a sufficient degree of functional efficiency. It is beyond the scope of this book to delve deep into critique of Boorse's view, but I deem this approach to be misguided. Instead, following Sander Werkhoven (2019) and Nordenfelt (2018), and developing their views (in light of my population health focus), I argue that health is an emergent property of complex systems, grounded in the capacities of those systems.

Whilst the health of an organism supervenes on the qualities of its parts, due to the complexity of organisms, the interactions of their physiological parts with one another and with their environments, and the ability of organisms to adapt to dysfunction at the part-level, the overall health of a biological system cannot be predicted simply by observing its parts, or indeed their contribution to survival, reproduction, or any other plausible goals, in isolation. I claim that health is a weakly emergent property, and accordingly a holistic approach to assessing the health of organisms must be adopted. Since the same principle can be applied to physiological parts (complex systems), organisms (complex systems), and to any population that properly qualifies as a complex system, this account has wide applicability. In this way, reifying health at the population level is not the mistake Jennings takes it to be.

In Sect. 2, I argue that Boorse's reductive approach to health fails to accommodate organisms as complex systems. In Sect. 3, I argue that health is best viewed as an emergent property of complex systems, and that any biological complex system is a suitable candidate for instantiating that property. Finally in Sect. 4, I present tentative criteria for what constitutes a complex system, demonstrate that at least some human populations qualify as complex systems, and how the health property can be understood in that context. I take the parsimony of the same account of health being applicable at all levels of biological organization to be an advantage of my view, and a disadvantage for those views unable to provide the same.

1.2 Reductive Accounts of Health

Whilst this is a book on philosophy of public health, and thus the primary matter of significance in this chapter is the nature of the health property as applied to the populations, I start by briefly considering reductive accounts of health at the level of the organism that fail to assign adequate weight to (weakly) emergent properties. The focus (as is so often the case in this field) will be on Boorse's BST. Once some major flaws in reductive analyses have been highlighted, I move to Werkhoven's holistic dispositionalist approach. This, I argue, avoids the problems of purely reductive accounts, and can be developed and applied at all levels of biological organization, from individual cells to the populations of countries. Although I take Werkhoven to provide interesting insights into how health can be measured, ultimately I argue it faces serious challenges—challenges that can be met by integrating the view with Nordenfelt's praxis-oriented concept of health (Nordenfelt 2018).

Boorse's Biostatistical Theory

The BST (Boorse 1997) comes in the form of four core tenets, and runs as follows:

1. The reference class is a natural class of organisms of uniform functional design; specifically, an age group of a sex of a species.
2. A normal function of a part or process within members of the reference class is a statistically typical contribution by it to their individual survival [or] reproduction.
3. Health in a member of the reference class is normal functional ability: the readiness of each internal part to perform all its normal functions on typical occasions with at least typical efficiency.

4. A disease [later, pathological condition] is a type of internal state which impairs health, i.e., reduces one or more functional abilities below typical efficiency (Boorse 1977, p. 562).

Boorse argues that health and disease are naturalist, value-free concepts. For him, the hallmark of disease is subnormal function, where the functional efficiency of a biological part is compared with biostatistically normal levels of efficiency for that organism's reference class (organisms of the same species, sex, and similar age). An organism is healthy only if every internal part "perform(s) all its normal functions on typical occasions with a least typical efficiency"; that is, if every internal part makes a biostatistically normal contribution towards the organism's individual survival or reproduction.

I will not consider the plethora of objections against the BST, many of which focus on drawing the line between normal and subnormal function. Let us assume for now that at the level of biological parts, Boorse is able to distinguish between healthy and diseased organs, tissues and cells. An individual cell *qua* physiological part is thus diseased once it no longer contributes to the natural goals of survival and reproduction with sufficient functional efficiency, however that is to be defined.

There is, however, a serious problem with this account of health at the level of the organism, even if Boorse's account of part-health is plausible. In humans, every day around 50 billion cells undergo programmed cell death (Kolb et al. 2017). Given that cells are physiological parts, and that Boorse defines health as *each internal* physiological part performing with at least typical functional efficiency, Boorse's reductive analysis entails that no human on Earth is healthy (Nordenfelt 1987). Boorse responds to objections of this kind as follows:

> At the pathologist's level of description, there is no paradox in calling one dead cell pathological, except, of course, in tissues like skin and mucosa whose normal function entails constant death and regeneration. One dead cell is just the ultimate in focal necrosis, one of pathology' s most common findings. Why would one dead neuron not be pathological? Is a dead neuron anormal neuron? Do dead neurons function normally? Since the neuron is a body part, in a tissue whose physiological function does not feature

> regular regeneration, it is not much more mysterious that its death is pathological than that the whole organism's death is pathological. (Boorse 1997, pp. 50–51)

On the face of it, Boorse just bites the bullet. He is interested in health and disease from the pathologist's perspective, not that of the clinician. It is simply true that all human beings have some degree of pathology. Perhaps some amendments to Boorse's third tenet could accommodate "normal functional ability" in an individual member of a reference class without requiring *all* their parts to exhibit normal functional efficiency, but Boorse's (1977) account fails to acknowledge that it is biologically normal to have many billions of physiological subsystems performing subnormally. If ordinary language use is any guide to the meaning of concepts (and it should be), then it cannot be the case that *nobody* is healthy.

Boorse's (1977) BST fails to account for the fact that humans, and indeed all other species of animal and plant, are complex systems. They are intricate systems of interdependent physiological parts that interact with one another, react to changes in the environment and to their relations with other physiological parts which often compensate for the dysfunction of others within that organism. Should one lose a kidney to disease, injury, or voluntary organ donation following a successful nephrectomy, the remaining healthy kidney will typically grow, compensating for the loss of the other and maintaining a healthy glomerular filtration rate (Lee et al. 2020). The health-status of an organism cannot, therefore, be established merely by looking for dysfunction within that organism's physiological subsystems considered in isolation, since an organism can often adapt so as to perform all its reference-class typical functions with a healthy degree of efficiency.

Following Werkhoven (2019) and Nordenfelt (2018), I claim the plausible alternative to a reductive approach of this kind, is to hold that the health of an organism can only be established holistically; that is, by considering its dispositions, capacities, or abilities as a complex system (see Sect. 4). The same approach can be applied at all levels of biological complexity.

Biological organisms are prime examples of complex systems. They are composed of many interacting parts at multiple levels of organization: cells, tissues, organs and organ-systems. They bear all the key markers of complex systems, including nonlinerarity, feedback-loops, self-organisation and adaptation (Kane and Higham 2015). Importantly, they instantiate (weakly) emergent properties.

> Weak emergence is not the kind of emergence, famously criticized by Hempel and Oppenheim, that involves ignorance about the causal web behind a system, and it is not a rejection of reductionism. On the contrary, weak emergence arises when a system's properties depend on just the combination of its parts and their organization. This is a context-sensitive form of reduction because a part's effect on the properties of the whole depends on the other parts (and any environmental factors) with which it interacts. (Bedau 2013)

Health cannot be reduced to the dysfunction of physiological parts considered in isolation. One must rather consider the emergent properties of complex biological systems; properties that supervene on the properties of systems at lower levels of complexity.

Health as a Secondary Property?

Alex Broadbent (2019a) claims that health is a secondary property; that is, health is value-free, but nonetheless subjective. At the level of physiological subsystems, health can easily be identified as a subjective notion on the grounds that medical practitioners choose where to draw the line between function and dysfunction. What counts as the "healthy range" for blood pressure in 25-year-old men is not an objective fact out there in nature to be discovered. Doctors and epidemiologists study large cohorts of patients and consider which levels are associated with increased risk of e.g. myocardial infarction. Where the experts draw the line between normal and abnormal function is thus not entirely arbitrary (it is based on practical considerations, often concerning the need for medical intervention), but it is nonetheless subjective.

The account of health I propose differs from Broadbent's insofar as Broadbent takes health to be a value-free property, and I do not. Whilst "health as a secondary property" might work if one is considering the theoretical notion of health (that used primarily by pathologists), I am interested in the concept that shapes public health policy. These concepts must be intrinsically tied to the needs and desires of those affected by the interventions.

1.3 Towards a Holistic Theory of Health

Werkhoven (2019) has argued for a dispositional theory of health. His holistic approach to organism health avoids the problems with reductive accounts highlighted earlier. He argues that health should be defined as the ratio of the organism's actual dispositions to the maximum dispositional set for a member of that organism's reference class. This definition provides a measure of the organism's degree of health, rather than identifying it as determinately healthy or unhealthy (I outline his analysis of these other concepts, shortly).

Like Boorse, Werkhoven takes reference classes to consist of age, sex, and species-type.[1] The maximum set of dispositions is to be determined empirically, by observing large numbers of members of each reference class, and identifying what capacities those members can in principle have.

> Health: Health is the ratio [the health ratio] of a living organism's dispositional set compared to the maximum dispositional set belonging to its reference class. (Werkhoven 2019, p. 934)

Crudely speaking, dispositional properties (dispositions) confer capacities on the particulars that instantiate them. Dispositions have stimulus conditions which, when met (and in the absence of finks or antidotes), result in their manifestation. The disposition 'solubility', for example, has

[1] Objections have been raised to these reference classes (Cooper 2002), but further discussion is beyond the scope of this chapter.

the stimulus condition of 'being mixed with water', and the manifestation of 'dissolving'. This process might be prevented if the water is already saturated, but *ceteris paribus* a soluble substance will always dissolve in water (Mumford 2004). Healthy humans have many thousands of capacities emerging from the dispositions of their physiological parts. A healthy 25-year-old human male has the capacity to run, lift weights, sleep, converse with their peers, breathe without difficulty, and so on. These capacities are weakly emergent properties, emerging from the dispositions of the individual's physiological parts. The more dispositions an organism has, Werkhoven argues, the healthier they are. For consistency, from this point I will focus on the emergent capacities (the things organisms are able to do), rather than the fundamental dispositions on which they supervene.

On the face of it, this view is largely consistent with our intuitions. Disease typically restricts what one is able to do. A severe chest infection will (at least temporarily) take away the patient's ability to do cardiovascular exercise, a broken ankle will take away the patient's capacities to walk, jump, run, cycle, and many other activities for which one requires two functioning ankles, and so on. Severe conditions have considerable effects on the patient's capacities: a patient in ICU has very few capacities compared to a healthy individual, and less severe conditions remove fewer capacities. Similarly, a patient with one kidney compensating for the loss of another has lost few capacities, so might still be considered healthy.

Jon Fuller (2018) has previously argued for a dispositional account of chronic diseases. He identifies a disease like epilepsy with the disposition to have seizures under certain stimulus conditions. Werkhoven's approach is somewhat different. Epilepsy would not be the disposition to have seizures (a gained disposition), but rather, the disposition to *lose* those capacities one loses whilst having seizures. The main benefit of adopting Werkhoven's approach over Fuller's, is that it is applicable to all diseases/reductions in health. For example, it is difficult to see how Fuller's approach could be applied to infectious diseases (something he doesn't claim to be able to do).

There are some further consequences of Werkhoven's account worth paying attention to, some more problematic than others. First, early-stage cancer will often not affect a patient's capacities in the short term. They can still run marathons, swim, and do all the things they could previously. Werkhoven thus concludes that it is not uncommon for patients to be both healthy *and* have a pathological condition. Health concerns the patient's current capacities, whereas the presence of a pathology reflects not just the patient's existing capacities, but their likely future capacities. I am happy to bite this bullet.

Second, some diseases *prima facie* confer dispositions on those they afflict, and according to Werkhoven's view, the more dispositions/capacities the healthier. The epilepsy example above demonstrates why this is problematic. Epilepsy confers the disposition to have seizures (or at least, the disposition to lose many normal functional abilities), but so long as the patient isn't having a seizure, this is not at the expense of any other dispositions or capacities. On the face of it, according to Werkhoven's account, unless in a state of seizure the epileptic is healthier than a non-epileptic with otherwise identical dispositions.

Third, Werkhoven places no restrictions on the kind of dispositions relevant to health. The dispositions conferring the capacity to read, for example, add to the health of a patient; and correspondingly, lacking that capacity counts as a health-deficit. Although medicine typically does not view illiteracy as a health problem (assuming it's not caused by poor eyesight or a mental disorder), Werkhoven is happy to see it as such. For him, then, not all health problems are medically treatable. Whilst this might be acceptable for a prescriptive account of health, it likely does not reflect the way health is or ever will be viewed by medical practitioners—the usual target of descriptive accounts of health and disease in the literature (this does not worry me, since (a) I, too, will provide a prescriptive account, and (b) public health need not invoke the same concept of health as clinicians).

Werkhoven's account faces further problems, however: he defines health in terms of the dispositions a patient instantiates, relative to "the maximal dispositional set". In this sense, his account is naturalist—it is value-free. The relevant dispositions are not chosen based on patient-values or the values of the patient's culture, since all dispositions count. But if we want an account of health that can be used, one needs to be able to count both the dispositions of the patient, and know how many dispositions are contained in the maximal dispositional set. I see no way to enumerate these dispositions. How many dispositions are required to pour a glass of water in circumstances S? Is it one (the capacity to pour a glass of water), or is it several (the disposition to extend one's arm in circumstances S, grip the bottle in circumstances S*, lift the bottle in circumstances S**, co-ordinate the bottle to the glass in circumstances S***, and so on). Or is the disposition to pour a glass of water in circumstances S an additional disposition to those finer-grained dispositions? Let us call this "the problem of enumeration".

The way around the problem of enumeration, I suggest, is to integrate Werkhoven's ratio-idea with something like Nordenfelt's Praxis-Oriented Concept of Health. Nordenfelt suggests that health is "the bodily and mental state of a person such that he or she has a second-order ability to realize his or her vital goals, given standard or otherwise accepted circumstances" (Nordenfelt 2018, p. 15), where the vital goals are

> goals that are inherent in all humans, and indeed… in all organisms. The vital goals include survival but they encompass much more…. a person's vital goals are the states of affairs that are necessary and jointly sufficient for his or her minimal long-term happiness. (Nordenfelt 2018, p. 14)

I propose a value-laden account whereby the capacities/abilities to be counted are identified based on those deemed necessary to promote "happiness" and "meaning in life" (I add "meaning in life" as a consideration for the vital goals for reasons I outline in detail in Chap. 6). In other words, a comprehensive, well-defined set of medically relevant capacities—those that contribute towards the vital goals—should be selected by medical and public health experts in a consultative process with their patients.

Not only must these capacities be identified, but they must be weighted relative to one another. Precisely how they are weighted is work beyond the scope of this chapter, but some capacities contribute more to achieving vital goals than others, and the more they contribute to the vital goals, the more weighting they deserve. Furthermore, the chosen capacities might be instantiated to varying degrees. Most adults have the capacity talk fluently and without difficulty, some people can talk to some degree, but struggle to do so for various reasons and in various ways, and others are mute. Patients can then be identified as either instantiating the specified capacities to degree X, or not instantiating these capacities, and their health measured accordingly.

This differs somewhat from Nordenfelt's view, first because I take the vital goals to reflect the capacities necessary for meaning in life, as well as happiness (see Chap. 6). And second, insofar as Nordenfelt takes the requirements of health to differ from one person to the next, since their vital goals can differ. The capacities one person needs for minimal long-term happiness can differ from the next. I nonetheless suggest, at least in the context of public health, that identifying a unique set of capacities against which the health of all individuals can be measured is a preferable option. A ubiquitously applicable set of capacities makes more sense from a pragmatic perspective. Nordenfelt himself grants that "most vital goals are shared by all people" (Nordenfelt 2018, p. 14)—it is the capacities necessary to achieve the universally shared vital goals that public health policy should focus on promoting. Note that this is not to say that the same intervention will help (or be needed by) all people achieve their vital goals. For example, wheelchair access might be a necessary intervention for all to obtain a particular vital goal, but not all will need to use it.

I suggest that this is true at all levels of biological complexity. When considering the health of a physiological subsystem, one should consider which of its capacities contribute to the vital goals of the organism, and to what extent. When considering the relevant capacities of a population (Sect. 4), one should consider which population-level capacities contribute to the vital goals of the population's members, and to what extent. Bearing this in mind, alongside my adoption of something akin to Werkhoven's health ratio, I define organism health as follows:

Organism Health: The ratio of an organism's weighted medically relevant capacities to the maximum set of weighted medically relevant capacities.

This modified version of the dispositional theory of health both avoids the absurd consequences of the reductionist approach (that there are no healthy human beings), and acts as a more suitable prescriptive account of health than Werkhoven's theory, stressing the role medicine should play in identifying those capacities relevant to health. Of course, what is considered a medically relevant capacity might change over time, but I consider that a virtue of the theory. What qualified as healthy in the fifteenth century may well not, today. And what counts as healthy today may well not in a century's time.

It's worth noting that the capacities an individual may have depends not only on their physiological health, but on the infrastructure around them, and on social and educational policies. For example, a deaf person's capacity to communicate with other people would be far less hindered, were everyone fluent in sign language. Similarly, someone paralysed from the hips down has more capacities in buildings equipped with wheelchair access. Given my account of organism health, one's health is deeply impacted by these things. Health is not just a function of one's physiology, but of one's surroundings, too.

This strategy provides a measure of health—the ratio of actual weighted capacities to those of the maximum set. However, as Werkhoven suggests, it admits of comparing the health states of different reference classes. One can compare the health of a 25-year-old human male with that of a 50-year-old human female, simply by comparing those ratios.

Andrew Schroeder (2013) argues that philosophers of medicine would be better off searching for a plausible comparative theory of health than looking for definitions of health and disease in absolute terms. The view I propose accommodates Schroeder's desideratum. If health is measured as a ratio, this ratio does not itself indicate whether the organism is *healthy* or not. A ratio indicating that the organism has only very few of the capacities included in the maximum set would be unhealthy, and an organism instantiating them all would be perfectly healthy, but if one is to identify the specific ratio demarcating the healthy from the unhealthy, then somewhere a line must be drawn. Werkhoven suggests the following solution:

> Healthy: X is healthy if and only if X's ratio (X's actual dispositional set compared to X's maximum possible dispositional set) is larger than the averaged ratio of a sufficiently large number of members of the relevant comparison class. (Werkhoven 2019, p. 935)

Although I agree that "healthy" needs to be a reference-class relative term, Werkhoven's definition is problematic. First, anyone below this average ratio could not be considered healthy, and we do not want to be committed to nearly half the population being unhealthy. Second, as Elselijn Kingma (2014) has pointed out, some populations are healthier than others, and this is problematic for any theory of health appealing to biostatistical averages to demarcate health and disease-states. During a highly contagious and harmful pandemic, for example, it's quite possible that the average health ratio could drop significantly. Thus, an organism with a health ratio of X could plausibly move from the unhealthy category (subnormal ratio) to the healthy category (normal/supernormal ratio), without any changes to their intrinsic properties/capacities. Health-status, on this view, is subject to radical Cambridge Changes (Guerrero 2010).

More broadly, this issue corresponds with the line-drawing problem identified by Peter Schwartz (2007) in his response to Boorse's Biostatistical Theory. Schwartz highlights that should Boorse wish to identify disease with part-dysfunction, and dysfunction with sub-normal (relative to the organism's reference class) function, he must somehow determine where the line demarcating normal from subnormal functional efficiency is to be drawn. Variations in both the average "absolute" health of a population, and variations in prevalence between different kinds of disease, make it impossible to pick a deviation from the mean that could be universally applied. Schwartz (2007) responds to this problem with his "Frequency and Negative Consequences Approach", concluding that the line demarcating health and disease should be drawn where the effects of the condition "significantly diminish the ability of a part or process in the organism, or of the overall organism, to carry out an activity that is generally standard in the species and has been for a long period of time" (Schwartz 2007). At the organism-level, this can reasonably be reinterpreted as "significantly reducing the capacities of the organism below what has been standard for the species for a long period of time" (Schwartz 2007, p. 379).

If Schwartz is looking for an objectivist solution to the line-drawing problem, then rather than solving it he has kicked the can down the road, introducing a further line-drawing problem. "The line" must now be drawn such that it identifies what counts as "significantly diminishing" the capacities of organisms below whatever is considered standard. So far as I can see, there is no plausible objectivist solution to this problem. That line must be drawn by medicine, relying on the subjective expert opinions of medical professionals. This reinforces my view that health is a subjectivist notion. Both the capacities relevant to health, their relative importance (the weightings), and the ratio required to be in a healthy-state, are mind-dependent, and should be determined by medical experts through a consultative process.[2]

Part-Health as an Emergent Property of Complex Systems

As we have seen, reductionists like Boorse take organism health to be reducible to the health of the organism's physiological parts. Just as humans and cows can be healthy, so can their livers and hearts. Whilst viewing organisms as complex systems allows one to make health assertions without appeal to the health of the individual's parts, it is nonetheless extremely important in the medical context to assess the health-states of physiological subsystems. After all, despite the health of an organism not being reducible to the health-states of its parts, its holistic state of health nonetheless supervenes on those parts. Furthermore, the successful treatment of unhealthy organisms will often require identifying an unhealthy physiological subsystem and returning it to a state of health. As I have already indicated, Boorse suggests that part-health is linked with statistically normal function. I argue, however, that the capacities approach I propose at the level of the organism is equally applicable at the level of physiological subsystems.

Organs, tissues, bodily fluids and cells are all complex systems. They have those same characteristics exemplified by all complex systems:

[2] This raises the issue of 'which experts'? A general practitioner might disagree with an oncologist. A psychiatrist might disagree with a pathologist, and so on. I do not have the space for a comprehensive discussion, but I am inclined to side with the expert judgment of general practitioners in the context of overall health judgments, and specialists in the context of part-health judgments. There will likely be disagreement even within specialists in their fields, but these matters can be debated until a near consensus is reached.

nonlinearity, feedback loops, self-organization and adaptation. Just as entire organisms have emergent properties that cannot be predicted by knowing and understanding the state of their parts alone, so biological cells have properties that emerge from the complex interactions of their parts and relations to other cells. As Avi Ma'ayan points out:

> ...the human cell is a complicated living natural machine. Cells that together compose our bodies are a prototypical example of a natural complex system that was evolved and optimized over billions of years. What partially makes human cells a typical complex system is that they are made of many different types of components with many copies of the same components, all working together, interacting in concert and in parallel to form a high-order functional entity that is a part of an organism. (Ma'ayan 2017, p. 6).

Given that physiological subsystems are complex systems, they are equally viable candidates for instantiating emergent properties as the organisms themselves. The kidney thus has the capacity to filter certain substances out of the blood, the heart has the capacity to beat at different rates under different conditions, and so on. The same account of health I propose at the organism level can thus be applied at the level of physiological parts. Medicine should identify the maximum set of weighted medically relevant capacities for physiological parts (for each reference class), determined by their contribution to the vital goals of the patient, and health is measured as the proportion of those capacities instantiated by each part relative to its respective maximum set.

Like health at the organism level, health at the level of the physiological part is a value-laden emergent property, since although the capacities they have are an objective biological fact, those deemed relevant to health by medical practitioners and researchers are ultimately a subjective choice driven by value-laden goals.

Varga's Contradicting Health-States Objection

It's worth noting an objection Somogy Varga has recently raised against health as a "gradable adjective" (those that admit of comparative analyses—X is healthier than Y). The objection explicitly targets negative concepts of health (health as the absence of disease), but in this context, he suggests that health as a gradable adjective generates contradictions. Consider the example he provides, below:

(a) A is unhealthy. He has celiac disease, an immune reaction to eating gluten, which can damage the intestinal lining, prevent absorption of some nutrients and cause diarrhea, fatigue, weight loss, and anemia. Fortunately, A never eats gluten
(b) B is healthy. Many of B's vitals (e.g., blood pressure, cholesterol, triglycerides, BMI) are, however, very close to being abnormal.
(c) A is healthier than B.

Consider also a similar comparison on the level of single organs.

(a') A is the unhealthy kidney of a 20-year-old. It is subject to a fully controlled kidney disease that reduces its functioning by 15%.
(b') B is the healthy kidney of a 92-year-old.
(c') A is healthier than B. (Varga, 2024, pp. 147–148)

Varga suggests that two sets of contradictions arise, here. For Varga, the 20-year-old with celiac disease should intuitively be seen as healthier than the technically healthy 92-year-old, despite the 20-year-old being deemed unhealthy, and the 92-year-old healthy. Similarly, despite the 20-year-old's kidney functioning subnormally, and coming out as "unhealthy" (on most accounts of health), that kidney should nonetheless be considered healthier than the "healthy" kidney of the 92-year-old.

The intuitions giving rise to both (c) and (c') arise (I assume) from equating degrees of health with degrees of functional efficiency. Varga states that "if both organs are up for donation and one has to choose the healthiest one, it is very likely that the choice will fall on [the 20-year-old's]" (Varga, 2024, p. 148). But if one takes the "reference class" condition to play a meaningful role in the (prescriptive) concept of health—as I do—one does not have to choose the healthiest kidney. Instead, one chooses that with the highest degree of functional efficiency. Context matters when determining both the health of individuals and the health of their organs, and the patient's reference class is central to that context.

Furthermore, Varga's contradictions rely on the identification of a "healthy" individual and an "unhealthy" kidney, respectively. As discussed previously, some of those (like Schroeder) advancing comparative theories of health (where "health" is a gradable adjective) would reject such notions. Regardless, relative to their respective reference classes, the 92-year-old *is* healthier than the 20-year-old, and the 92-year-old's kidney *is* healthier than that of the 20-year-old.

1.4 Healthy Populations?

Animal (Including Human) Populations as Complex Systems

Thus far I have argued that reductivist accounts of health (that do not consider emergent properties) should be rejected in favour of a holistic, capacities-based account. Health can be viewed as an emergent property of both organisms and their physiological parts, since both organisms and their parts constitute complex systems. In this section, I argue that populations, too, qualify as complex systems, capable of instantiating the health property.

The idea that the "public" in public health (and the various subpopulations within this public) can be reified in such a way that this property attribution is coherent, is a contentious matter. Richard Mohr argues that:

> No literal sense exists in which there could be such a thing as a public health. To say the public has a health is like saying the number seven has a color: such a thing cannot have such a property. You have health or you lack it and I have health or lack it, because we each have a body with organs that function or do not function. But the public, an aggregate of persons

> similarly disposed as persons, has no such body of organs with functions which work or fail. (Mohr 1987, p. 96)

Like Jennings, Mohr claims that the public is not the kind of entity that can instantiate properties—certainly not a property like health. However, his argument is not persuasive for at least two reasons: first, it is widely accepted in medicine that organs can be healthy or unhealthy. It is quite normal to talk of e.g., cardiovascular or heart health. Yet hearts, as organs, do not themselves have "a body with organs". If we accept the meaningfulness of "heart health" (it seems perfectly meaningful to me), having a body with organs cannot be a prerequisite of "having health".

Second, Mohr assumes that the public is a mere "aggregate of persons"—but this is at least questionable. As Elodie Giroux argues:

> Recognizing the importance of the population level of analysis has led certain epidemiologists to give it back its central place in the discipline and to defend the necessity of a change of paradigm… The population is considered to be a pertinent level of organization in itself, both for measurements and for analysis and inference. For these epidemiologists, it is about returning to social medicine as a source of inspiration. (Giroux 2021, p. 13)

Just as human bodies are complex systems of interdependent physiological parts (interacting with their microbiome(s) and broader social environments), so the public comprises interdependent members of populations. The target of public health is typically not an arbitrary class of individuals (for example, a single randomly selected person from every country in the world), but a class of individuals (a population) working together towards shared goals, depending on one another, compensating for one another in a variety of ways, and so on. In this way, populations comprise a complex system, able to instantiate emergent properties that cannot be predicted by examining its component parts independently of one another.

I make a more substantive case for this, shortly, but to establish the *prima facie* plausibility of populations instantiating health properties, let us consider the curious case of Colony Collapse Disorder (CCD) in honeybees.

Colony Collapse Disorder

Honeybees, which play an important role in human health through plant pollination, honey production and its associated economic impact, are facing a crisis. There is growing concern that the drastic global rise in CCD will result in severely depleted bee populations, which could have devastating consequences not only for beekeepers (and their bees), but for the environment more generally. As the name suggests, CCD is not a disorder of an individual bee. It is a disorder of the colony, whereby the majority of worker bees in a colony leave the hive and do not return. They abandon the queen bee, the honey they have produced, and the juvenile bees. This quickly results in the collapse of the colony.

Fabrice Requier, in his 2019 paper "Bee colony health indicators, synthesis and future directions", writes that:

> Honeybee colonies can be assimilated to a complex system for which survival depends on its individual quality, its adaptive capacity and its threshold of resilience to pressures. (Requier 2019, p. 1)

Beekeepers, when they speak of the health of their colony, are not speaking metaphorically. CCD is a real disorder, and one that applies to the colony (the collective), not to the individual bees, which, despite abandoning the hive, may themselves suffer from no pathological conditions as individuals. The health deficit of the colony is thus an emergent property, not predictable by examining the health of individual bees in isolation.

One might question whether the 'health' property, as attributed to a bee colony, is the very same property as that one attributes to the individual bee. But the fact that an analysis of "colony health" will differ in some ways to that of "individual bee health" does not imply the term is being used either metaphorically or incorrectly. If bee colonies can truthfully be described as instantiating health properties in virtue of their comprising complex systems, there is good reason to believe the same is true of at least some human populations (Smart 2023a).

Human Populations as Complex Systems[3]

Drawing on David Fishner and Jonathan Pruitt, I (with Herkulaas Combrink) have argued elsewhere that human populations plausibly comprise complex systems capable of instantiating emergent properties (Smart and Combrink 2022). Fishner and Pruitt highlight eight characteristics of complex systems in the context of animal populations:

Hierarchy: "Hierarchy refers to cases where systems exhibit structural properties at multiple organizational levels. More specifically, a complex system can be arranged in a series of nested groups, where connections are more frequent within than between neighboring groups, and that nestedness can extend to multiple levels" (Fisher and Pruitt 2020, p. 2).

Human populations clearly instantiate 'hierarchy' in this sense. Societies are structured in such a way that members of small communities interact with one another more frequently than members of neighboring communities, and although interactions with distant communities occur, such interactions are even less frequent. This feature of human populations played a key role in certain non-pharmaceutical interventions in the recent COVID-19 pandemic. In South Africa, for example, where a risk-adjusted mitigation strategy was imposed, the strictest form of lockdown aimed to minimize human-interactions at even the local community level, by keeping everyone at home (except for essential services). As lockdown restrictions were relaxed, movement within one's community was permitted, but traveling to communities in other provinces remained off limits (Stiegler and Bouchard 2020).

Heterogeneity: "Complex systems can be made up of interacting components which are heterogeneous, in that they differ in their behavior, location, history, or other properties." (Fisher and Pruitt 2020, p. 4).

This is perhaps more true of human populations than any other animal species. The many different professions in (at least first world) human populations are indicative of the vast number of distinct functional roles adults can play in society, and in addition, a relatively large proportion of human populations play little functional role, at least in terms of economic activity and food production, compared with most animal species

[3] Permissions from JECP.

(children typically don't begin to work until at least 16, and most adults retire before 67).

Self-organization: "Self-organization is a property of many kinds of systems, both living and non-living, including animal populations. If a system is self-organized, then interactions between individual units of the system… combine to give emergent properties at higher levels of organization" (Fisher and Pruitt 2020, p. 5).

Again, this is true of human populations. Interactions between individuals give rise to healthcare systems, education systems, and the entire global economy. As Elodie Giroux (2021) highlights, Georges Canguilhem has argued that there is no self-organization and internal normativity in human populations, since "the normativity is not biological and internal but social and external"[4] (Canguilhem 1988). Whilst I might accept the premise of this (despite there being clear biological components in the familial context—mothers breastfeeding children, and so forth), I do not accept the conclusion. I see no reason to assume that self-organization and normativity must be either biological or internal.

Openness: "Energy, information, and disturbances can alter complex systems from beyond the system boundaries… Ecosystems, networks of neurones, electrical networks such as the Internet and weather systems are all influenced by external inputs… Animal populations too exhibit a high degree of openness, but their degree of openness may vary situationally or across species" (Fisher and Pruitt 2020, p. 5).

Human populations are of course subject to disturbances that alter their operations. Examples are not difficult to find, but the COVID-19 pandemic demonstrates just how "open" the human population, as a complex system, is.

Memory: "Information about the past may be retained in a complex system, which can influence how the complex system behaves in the future. This is often referred to as system's "memory"" (Fisher and Pruitt 2020, p. 5).

The mere fact that this book is being written is demonstrative of memory within the human population as a complex system. Perhaps more

[4] Private correspondence with Elodie Giroux. My thanks to her for this comment.

noticeably, though, generation after generation have transformed their environment for those who stand to inherit it.

Nonlinearity: "A key aspect of complex systems is that changes often show nonlinear trends, so that outputs from the system are disproportionate to inputs" (Fisher and Pruitt 2020, p. 7).

Nonlinearity is observable in many aspects of human populations, including the social arena. For example, a phenomenon known as "quorum responses" has been observed, whereby the vast majority of individuals rapidly reach a consensus decision, once a sufficient number of other individuals have made it (Seeley and Visscher 2003).

Adaptation: "Adaptation refers to changes in the behavior of a complex system in response to changes in outside influence" (Fisher and Pruitt 2020, p. 8).

Clearly human populations are remarkably adaptable. We live in some of the hottest and coldest climates in the world, can adapt to both very wet and very dry conditions, and put measures in place to mitigate the effects of pandemics.

Uncertainty: "Complex systems are often characterized by low predictability. This low predictability can be caused by systems' sensitivity to initial conditions or through the difficulty of predicting emergent phenomena" (Fisher and Pruitt 2020, p. 9).

Finally, it would be hard to argue for the predictability of human behaviour. Who could have known in 2018 that the global economy would come to a complete standstill in 2 years' time, with social distancing and even self-isolation becoming a normal part of everyday life?

These eight criteria are all exemplified by human populations, so I consider there to be a good case for understanding human populations as complex systems—and further, that this has important implications for understanding health at this level of biological organization. As complex systems, human populations are suitable candidates for instantiating emergent properties (Ladyman et al. 2013)—the health property, I claim, stands among them.

Health as an Emergent Property of Populations

Now that I have established that human populations are capable of instantiating emergent properties as a collective (in virtue of being genuine complex systems), and have provided *prima facie* motivation on the grounds that other animal populations (honeybees) are already viewed as collectively instantiating health/disease properties, I can progress to outlining what it might mean to measure the health of populations.

Just as health is an emergent property of organisms and their biological parts, so it can be viewed as an emergent property of populations; furthermore, just as (I claim) this property should be characterized in terms of capacities at the lowest levels of biological organization (e.g., individual cells), so it should be at the highest (populations). In this section, I provide two possible interpretations: a broad interpretation, and a narrow interpretation. Although the narrow account arguably provides the measure of population health those working in public health would be most interested in, the broad interpretation allows health researchers and policymakers to focus more on wider social justice/egalitarian issues, such as dealing with poverty and inequality. Thus, despite the narrow account being more applicable to public health institutions, it is not necessarily the account policymakers at government level should pay the most attention to.

The capacities-based measure of population health I propose is functionally similar to my account of *Organism Health* (above). First, one establishes the maximum relevant set of capacities for the population. This can be done with both a broad and narrow understanding of public health. On the narrow understanding, the focus is on areas typically deemed relevant to the field of public health as traditionally understood—e.g., capacities deemed relevant to medical care/preventative medicine, clean water, sanitation, and so forth—in short, interventions that affect human physiological health. On the broader understanding, one can include capacities relevant to population health understood as improving the wellbeing of populations more generally. This might include capacities relevant to education, freedom of speech, freedom of movement, and political engagement (see Chaps. 2 and 6). Second, one contrasts the maximum relevant set of weighted capacities with the actual capacities of a specific population, to form a public health ratio. The higher the ratio, the healthier the population.

A population has capacities in virtue of the collaborative efforts, skills, resources of its members, and of the state at large. These capacities are thus emergent properties of the population as a complex system. A population might have the capacity to effectively deal with a serious epidemic (the collaborative work of a large number of interdependent individuals), grow economies, provide clean water and sanitation, and so on.

Within the global population of humans (arguably itself a complex system), many subsets of this population comprise legitimate complex systems. Whilst some public health interventions might have a global reach (interventions on e.g., climate change might count among those), most are more restricted. A rational comparative measure of the health of the South African population (its public health ratio) requires the capacities of the South African population to be measured against the maximum set of capacities for nation states. In short, like with physiological subsystems and organisms, suitable reference classes must be identified in order to make comparative health judgements.

Of course, the maximum set of capacities for human populations changes over time. In 1650, no human population could offer a large-scale immunization programmes. That is no longer true, and the capacity to immunize against various diseases should be included in the maximum set. Since the potential (and actual) capacities of human populations are forever improving, when comparing the health of past populations with that of present populations, we are left with a dilemma: either time-index the public health ratio so that the health of a population in the year 1850 is measured against the maximum set of capacities for human populations in 1850, or calculate the public health ratio for all time periods relative to the maximum set of capacities at the present moment. If we choose the latter option, the public health ratios of past populations are forever decreasing. If we choose the former, we must accept that some populations in the distant past may have been significantly healthier than many contemporary populations, even though the life expectancy of the average person was significantly lower, and child mortality rates significantly higher. It seems intuitive that present-day populations are healthier than past populations, and so the latter option seems preferable. It enables us to measure population health, whilst acknowledging that future generations will (hopefully) consider all early twenty-first century human populations relatively unhealthy.

Any human population that qualifies as a complex system can instantiate the health property. Thus, although a class of randomly selected individuals from different countries will not satisfy conditions such as nonlinearity and feedback loops (and therefore not count as a complex system), the class of individuals living in South Africa would. Population health interventions often focus on well-specified, fairly narrowly defined and (and as a consequence) smaller populations. For example, it may consider ways of improving the mental health of women who have recently given birth. Whether these smaller populations comprise a genuine complex systems will differ from case to case—often they will not.

Many public health interventions, on the other hand, focus on broader populations—the population of a nation state, for example. Everyone living in South Africa is affected by the activities of its other residents. Many pay taxes to the central government, and this government uses those funds to pay for education, healthcare, infrastructure development, and so on. Some residents farm, and nearly all residents eat South African farm produce. The lives of South Africans, no matter how separated on the face of it, are interconnected in a variety of ways such that together, emergent properties arise. As I have argued, these include properties such as the capacity to build infrastructure and mitigate against infectious diseases. For both the broad and narrow interpretations of population health, these emergent capacities (whatever capacities are identified as relevant to public health) would determine the health of the population.

From the above, we can formulate the following definition of Population Health:

Population Health: the ratio of a qualifying (in virtue of being a complex system) population's (relevant) weighted capacities compared to the maximum set of (relevant) weighted capacities belonging to its reference class.

This, like *Organism Health*, does not tell us what counts as "healthy". It merely provides the yardstick by which health is to be (comparatively) measured. At the organism level, Werkhoven suggests that "healthy" organisms are those with a health ratio greater than the average ratio of those within its reference class. I demonstrated this to be problematic, first on the grounds that this approach is likely to identify too many organisms as unhealthy, and second on the grounds that it does not accommodate "unhealthy populations". For the same reasons (it's quite possible for the majority of populations within a reference class to be unhealthy), I diverge from Werkhoven's appeal to statistical averages in determining the requirements for populations to be deemed healthy.

If one must classify populations as healthy or unhealthy, I contend that the subjective opinions of those working in public health are used to "draw the line" between healthy and unhealthy health ratios at the population level. Just as medicine makes informed choices regarding what constitutes the "normal range" of healthy blood pressure, so public health stakeholders might make informed decisions concerning a "healthy" public health ratio.

Choosing the Relevant Capacities

In Chap. 2 I discuss the goal of public health in depth, but crudely speaking, the goal of public health is (at least in part) to improve the health of the public. What this amounts to, of course, is dependent on how one construes the health of the public, and this can be (for want of a better word) manipulated by choosing those metrics by which the health of the public is assessed. In our context, that means through the selection of those capacities that together comprise the maximum set of capacities against which the health of individual populations is measured.

Some capacities are quite naturally linked to public health. The capacity of a population to deal with epidemics, provide clean water, sanitation, build and operate hospitals, provide immunizations, and so on. But in order to place a focus on poverty and inequality, on the broad interpretation of population health one might further include the capacity for social mobility; that is, the capacities of the poorest among the population to climb out of poverty into the middle class.

Precisely which capacities are to be included, however, is a subjective choice, determined by the values of society. Governments and other stakeholders can thus choose which capacities to include and exclude as relevant to public health based on the values (including ethical values) of society, and shape their public health policy based on these. In Chap. 6 on capacities-based principlism (a new framework for public health ethics), I suggest that John Rawls's theory of justice (Rawls 1971). Nussbaum's (2011) Capabilities Approach to human dignity, and Sridhar Venkatapuram's (2013) Capabilities Approach to health can provide useful guidance on which capacities could be included in this account, but like values in general, I maintain that these are subject to change, and may differ in specifics from one cultural context to the next.

1.5 Conclusions

In this chapter I have argued in favour of a capacities account of health at all levels of biological organization. Health should be viewed as an emergent property of complex systems, applicable as much to populations as it is to individual organisms and their physiological parts. I first rejected the account of organism-health provided by Boorse, demonstrating that a holistic account of health is necessary at the organism level. Drawing on and developing Werkhoven's dispositional account of health and Nordenfelt's praxis-oriented concept of health, I proposed a capacities-based theory at both the organism and part-level, whereby the health of an organism (or its parts) is the ratio of their medically relevant capacities to those of the maximum set of capacities for their reference class.

I further demonstrated that the human populations with which public health is concerned comprise genuine complex systems, and thus qualify for emergent property attribution. The health of a population is one such property, and can be determined by the ratio of its public health-relevant capacities to those of the maximum set of relevant capacities for its reference class. This admits of comparing the health of different human populations. Whether a population is deemed "healthy" or not, however, will depend on the standards set by the relevant experts. There is no mind-independent line to be drawn demarcating the healthy and unhealthy, regardless of the level of biological organization (cell, organ, organism, population).

2

The Goal of Public Health

2.1 Outline

Little can be achieved in the domain of public health without first identifying its goals. During the COVID-19 pandemic, the phrase "following the science" was regularly used by politicians from both the global north and global south in order to justify draconian public health interventions (Stevens 2020). But what, precisely, does "following the science" mean? Applied sciences like public health do not operate in a vacuum. Whereas an epidemiologist might be able to explain and/or describe the distribution and determinants of disease, for example, this alone has no implications on policymaking. Before public health policy is established, policymakers must first agree on the goals of public health interventions. Once these goals have been identified, one can use the sciences (very broadly construed, to include social sciences such as economics, politics, anthropology, sociology and psychology, as well as medicine and epidemiology) to make reasonable predictions regarding how these goals can best be achieved.

In South Africa, the national government's oft-repeated goal regarding the COVID-19 interventions was to "flatten the curve"—crudely

B. Smart, *The Philosophy of Public Health*,
https://doi.org/10.1007/978-3-031-98804-2_2

speaking, this was shorthand for reducing the basic reproduction number (or R-naught) of the virus below 1.0 (Adams 2020). The United Kingdom (UK) adopted the slogan "Save Our NHS"—in 2020 the UK's National Health Service, like nearly all healthcare systems worldwide, was massively overburdened with patients suffering from COVID-19. Like South Africa, then, the primary (if not the only) public health goal espoused by politicians in the UK was to reduce the direct burden of the virus. But of course, those interventions, even if effective, were always going to have significant public health implications beyond the effects of the virus itself, both in the short and long term.

I argued in Chap. 1 that the health of a population should be measured in terms of its capacities. Sustained lockdowns severely affect the capacities of a population, not only in their effects on the physical and mental health of those individuals comprising that population, but predominantly through the inability of populations to function normally in lockdown conditions. Businesses and indeed entire economies struggled during COVID lockdowns, globally. Infrastructure could not be constructed or properly maintained, and education was severely affected at all levels (Smart et al. 2021). In the years that followed the COVID-19 outbreak, due (at least in part) to the enormous sums of money spent on COVID relief packages, the global money supply soared, inflation rose, and interest rates spiked putting enormous pressure on ordinary people, but especially the poor.

Of course, where the effect of an epidemic is sufficiently severe, and lockdown is likely to be an effective intervention against a highly transmissible and very deadly pathogen, harsh lockdown conditions can be warranted on the grounds that lesser interventions would result in worse overall outcomes. However, I have argued (with colleagues) elsewhere that in at least some countries (including South Africa), the severity of the lockdown in 2020 was misguided (Smart et al. 2021).

Given the age-distribution of the country (in 2020 South Africa had an median age of 27 and relatively few people over 65, and COVID-19 predominantly severely affected only the elderly), and given the high-density township living conditions of the majority of the population, there was always a high likelihood that the lockdown (where, crudely, citizens were initially unable to leave their homes except for groceries and medical treatment) would fail; that is, the direct and indirect population health consequences of hard lockdown were never likely to be worth enduring for whatever health benefit it might have. "Flattening the curve" is not a legitimate public health goal; at best, it is a means to an end—to reduce the country's excess deaths. But this goal alone ignores all the short-term and long-term indirect consequences of the intervention, and just as no drug is approved without consideration of both its effectiveness and side effects, so no public health intervention should be implemented without due consideration of its probable effectiveness, and importantly, its adverse consequences.[1]

To make good public health policy decisions, and to make sense of "following the science", a clear understanding of the goal of public health is necessary. This chapter considers what the goal of public health should be, concluding that it should be to improve the population's public health ratio by maximizing the capacities deemed relevant to public health (in the broad sense discussed in Chap. 1). Any public health policy maker with this goal in mind must pay as much attention to the capacities public health interventions sacrifice, as it does to those they promote.

In this chapter, drawing primarily on Bengt Brülde (Brülde 2011) and Christian Munthe (Munthe 2008), I outline various attempts at capturing the goal of public health. I apply my interpretation of health at both the individual and population levels to these accounts, and consider how they might address health inequalities. I conclude that the goal of public health should be to promote those emergent capacities of populations (as complex systems) that maximally improve the opportunities for individuals (the population's members) to be/stay in good health.

2.2 The Traditional Interpretation

The "traditional goal of public health" (the traditional interpretation) is simply to improve population health. Population health is generally ill-defined, and as I discussed in Chap. 1, often considered at best a metaphorical notion. Munthe claims that "population health in this context is the idea of an aggregate of individual health levels, states, trends etc., and

[1] Further discussion of South Africa's response to the COVID-19 pandemic can be found in Chap. 3.

thus the traditional interpretation is consequentialist in its basic construction" (Munthe 2008, p. 40). On the face of it, the traditional goal gives rise to some interesting conflicts with additional possible goals of public health, some of which have gained traction in the last 50 years or so; in particular, those pertaining to health inequalities and autonomy.

Given the choice between two public health interventions: A and B, where A raises the aggregate individual health levels, states, trends, etc. more than B, but increases health inequalities within the population at large, and B improves the individual health levels, states, trends, etc. of the disadvantaged, but fails to improve the overall aggregate so much as intervention A, which should we choose? It's likely that those who take egalitarian issues seriously will *ceteris paribus* opt for B.

I argue in this chapter that the capacities approach to measuring public health enables public health policymakers to select the appropriate interventions to both improve population health (from a biomedical perspective) and reduce public health inequalities. First, however, I explore the traditional interpretation in more detail, integrating this with the notion of public health-ratios considered in Chap. 1.

Aggregating Health: The HALEs Approach

Bengt Brülde suggests, with some modifications, that public health should aim to maximize Healthy Life Expectancy (HALEs). The standard HALEs approach provides one way of quantifying the traditional interpretation, concluding that the goal of public health is to maximize the number of years people live in "full health". Naturally, relatively few people live in what might be called "perfect health" (at least not for very long), so Brülde presents a number of interpretative options: first (one that he ultimately rejects), that "each improvement in health of a certain magnitude is equally valuable (from a public health perspective), regardless of where on the scale it occurs" (Brülde 2011, p. 27).

Brülde goes on to consider various analyses of health in individuals, including Jerome Wakefield's hybrid account (Wakefield 1992) and Christopher Boorse's biostatistical theory (Boorse 1977). Wakefield, focusing on mental disorders, argues that disorders have both an evaluative and an explanatory (non value-laden) criteria. A disease, for Wakefield, must be considered a bad thing to have by the patient's cultural standards (the value criterion), and be the result of some physiological dysfunction (the explanatory criterion—Wakefield prefers evolutionary accounts of dysfunction, whereby dysfunction is failure to perform the function that best explains the trait's presence in the organism). Boorse, on the other hand, offers what he takes to be a naturalist, objectivist perspective. Crudely speaking, Boorse argues that disease is subnormal part function relative to the organism's reference class (see Chap. 1).

It is beyond the scope of this chapter to go deep into the arguments against these views, but Brülde concludes that none of the existing analyses provide adequate necessary and sufficient conditions for the concept of disease, and that some family resemblance analysis is probably required. He does not, however, consider Werkhoven's dispositional analysis or Nordenfelt's praxis-oriented account of health (excusable, given that they were written years after Brülde's paper was published), some aspects of which I explicitly endorse for all biological complex systems (see Chap. 1).

If, as I suggest, one adopts the capacities approach to the health of complex systems (including individual organisms), the HALEs approach suggests that the goal of public health is to maximize the relevant capacities of individuals within a population.

In order to fully understand how this approach might operate, one must be explicit about what "aggregating" means in the context of aggregating individual health/dispositional states. As Munthe (2008) notes, this approach is broadly consequentialist in nature, and one can draw on the consequentialism literature to reveal possible interpretations. First, one might simply take aggregation to be the total sum of all the capacities of the individuals, such that when two people instantiate the same capacity (say, the capacity to run), these count as two capacities. The aim of public health under the traditional interpretation (ignoring, for now, the emergent capacities of the collective), would thus be to maximize the health of the public by maximizing the sum of all the individuals' capacities. Let us call this the "Basic Enumeration Strategy" (BES).

One apparent trouble with this approach emerges from the fact that it is closely related to Derek Parfit's *Impersonal Total Principle*:

> *The Impersonal Total Principle:* other things being equal, the best possible outcome is the one in which there would be the greatest quantity of whatever makes life worth living. (Parfit 1984, p. 387)

Good health, identifiable in terms of capacities, is certainly one of the things that makes life worth living. But the impersonal total principle generates what Parfit aptly coined "The Repugnant Conclusion":

> *The Repugnant Conclusion:* for any possible population of at least ten billion people, all with a very high quality of life, there must be some much larger imaginable population whose existence, if other things are equal, would be better, even though its members have lives that are barely worth living. (Parfit 1984, p. 388)

The repugnant conclusion is just as applicable to the BES under the HALEs approach as it is to the consequentialist's impersonal total principle. On the face of it, BES implies that it is (or at least could be) better to have a population of a hundred billion people with relatively few capacities, than a population of ten billion people living in very good health. Keeping as many people alive for as long as possible, regardless of their health state, would indeed be a repugnant conclusion—one that might suggest the ban on contraceptives mentioned earlier as an effective public health intervention. Partly for this reason, in Chap. 5 I dismiss welfarist (total) utilitarian approaches to public health ethics.

2.3 Health Inequalities and the Social Determinants of Health

In the introduction to this chapter, I suggested that goals over and above the improvement of individuals' health states are now being taken seriously; perhaps most notably, (1) addressing health inequalities (Woodward and Kawachi 2000), and (2) respecting the autonomy of the individuals involved (Buchanan 2008). It is common for these additional goals to conflict with the traditional goal. A vaccine mandate during a pandemic would, whilst hopefully being an effective public health intervention, reducing the risk of succumbing to the disease in question, undermine the autonomy of those unwilling to take it. Similarly, the easiest and *prima facie* most effective public health interventions to implement will often target those who already have access to good service delivery and healthcare facilities (Munthe 2008), and not those most in need (more on this in Chap. 5).

Munthe claims that integrating the autonomy desideratum means "that even a perfect score in terms of this goal is logically and conceptually compatible with a very low level of population health" (Munthe 2008, p. 43). This follows, because if the goal of public health is to "create societal prerequisites for good health on equal terms for the entire population… *if they want to*[2]" (Munthe 2008, p. 42), then individuals can always choose not to take advantage of the healthcare opportunities (more on autonomy in Sect. 2.4).

The capacity to provide high quality healthcare to everyone would be an emergent property of the population, and can be present irrespective of uptake. Of course, the capacities of the individuals comprising that population would (overall) likely be less affected by a disease should they choose to e.g., take the vaccine, but the capacity of the population (typically with government intervention) to provide the vaccines alone contributes to population health as a collective, according to the capacities approach (see Chap. 1).

Brülde's Moderated HALEs Approach

For now, focusing on health inequalities more generally, it seems right to suggest that an improvement to the health state of someone in poor health is more valuable than an improvement of the same magnitude to someone in excellent health. This is analogous to the difference between giving someone living in poverty USD1000, and giving a billionaire USD1000. That amount of money makes no tangible difference to the billionaire, but could make a significant difference to someone living in poverty. Similarly, providing those in poor health with the care they

[2] My emphasis.

require to regain certain basic capacities is arguably far more valuable than endowing those with supernormal capacities with additional ones. The BES with HALEs fails to address these differences.

Brülde attempts to address this problem by introducing a weighted system, such that the "better a person's health is, the less is the value of a certain improvement, that is, the marginal value of health is diminishing" (Brülde 2011, p. 28).

As Brülde explains: "We represent each life graphically, in the form of a curve. The number of weighted life years are still represented on the x-axis, but we no longer measure people's health states on the y-axis. The y-axis is no longer a straightforward heath scale, but a "health value scale" that consists of "weighted health units". It is the area below this curve that we should try to maximize, that is, weighted HALEs" (Brülde 2011, p. 28).

Brülde's graph indicates that the worse an individual's health is, the more impact each degree of improved health has on the area under the graph. The weighted life years on the x-axis further suggest that extending life in relatively young people is more important, from a public health perspective, than extending life in the elderly. In this way, Brülde is able to accommodate the priority public health should place on health inequalities, placing a focus on those with low life expectancy and low individual degrees of health.

Whilst Brülde's Moderated HALEs Model has its advantages over the traditional view, which fails altogether to prioritize those in poor health and thus to address any health inequalities, in my opinion it still fails to encapsulate the complete picture of public health. Brülde states that "there are abilities (such as the ability to read or to swim) that have nothing to do with health" (Brülde 2011, p. 34), and whilst I agree that the ability to read or to swim has nothing to do with medicine, the ability to swim and read *are* relevant to public health more broadly construed. The ability to swim and read are capacities that help people lead more fulfilling and meaningful lives. Not only that, but the ability to swim can be a life-saving capacity, and the ability to read is typically a necessary condition of earning a stable income to keep one out of poverty, and is associated with better health outcomes (Nutbeam 2008). So, although teaching children (or indeed adults) to swim may not be a medical intervention, it could certainly be viewed as a public health intervention (see Chap. 6). This kind of example is hardly unusual: ensuring the public has access to clean water is a classic public health intervention, but no medical intervention is involved.

The Social Determinants of Health

In 1978, Michael Marmot *et al* published their findings from the Whitehall study of British civil servants (Marmot et al. 1978). This study set out to identify the relationship between employment status and risk of death. It was discovered that "the lower the grade of employment, the higher the mortality rate" (Marmot 2023, p. 207). Interestingly, the correlation goes far beyond the obvious link between poverty and poor health outcomes. Even those civil servants somewhere in the middle of the employment grades, whom all received sufficient income to provide adequate nutrition for themselves and their families, receive good quality healthcare, and so on, had worse health outcomes than their seniors. This outcome was somewhat surprising, given the long-held belief that the high-stress associated with higher-grade employment status increases one's risk of cardiovascular disease. The Whitehall study completely contradicted this, showing the inverse: the lower the employment grade (with less responsibility and correspondingly lower stress), the higher the risk of cardiovascular disease.

Karasek and Theorell (1990) and later Marmot provide us with an explanation: risk of heart disease is not "just demand… but also how much control one had over the work" (Marmot 2023, p. 210); that is, low control over one's work turned out to be a good predictor of the incidence of heart disease, and, "statistically contributed to the social gradient in heart disease" (Marmot 2023, p. 210). This ultimately led Marmot to develop a "general theory of empowerment as underlying global health inequalities"—a strategy that aligns well with a capacities approach to measuring population health. After all, to empower citizens just is to endow them with further capacities.

Marmot was later asked by the British government to provide public health recommendations based on his findings. The following six policy objectives were proposed in what became known as "The Marmot Review":

- Give every child the best start in life
- [Empower citizens through] education and life-long learning
- [Improve] employment and working conditions
- Ensure everyone has at least the minimum income necessary for a healthy life
- Healthy and sustainable places in which to live and work
- Taking a social determinants approach to prevention. (Marmot 2010, p.15)

It is worth noting that these recommendations are context-specific: they apply to England post-2010. Few people in England, if any, struggle to find access to clean water. Infectious diseases common in some parts of the developing world, such as HIV/AIDS and tuberculosis, are relatively rare, with cardiovascular diseases and Dementia and Alzheimers disease being the leading cause of death in 2023 (Office for National Statistics 2023). Bearing that in mind, these recommendations would nonetheless be exportable to other contexts, including the developing world (although the developing world typically has extra work to do, and perhaps to prioritize, in providing adequate infrastructure and dealing with infectious diseases). Noticeably, each one serves to improve the capacities of either the individuals comprising the population, those of the population as a collective, or both.

I cannot do justice to Marmot's recommendations, here, but since "giving every child the best start in life" is somewhat vague, it warrants further discussion. Central to this recommendation is providing children with high quality nutrition and "good parenting" (specifically referring to "reading to children"). Both (good nutrition and reading to children) are correlated with affluence and inversely correlated with economic deprivation.

The more income a family receives, the easier it is to provide children with an adequate supply of nutritious food. It is well established that low-income households tend to eat less healthily, in large part because healthier foods tend to be more expensive and/or harder to access (Harrison et al. 2010). Furthermore, whilst, as Marmot notes, the political right tend to blame the parents of deprived children for the poor parenting they receive (e.g., a failure to regularly read or even talk to young children), the "poor parenting" is itself a consequence of the deprived families' living conditions. Marmot thus recommends two complimentary strategies: (1) to address deprivation and inequality, and (2) to provide support for parents and families. Improving both child-nutrition and parenting would significantly help early childhood development, improving their cognitive, social, and behavioral skills, in turn providing them with the capacities required to learn effectively at school.

Similar comments can be made about "education and lifelong learning". The primary goal of education is to equip citizens with the capacities required to become productive members of society. If governments want to improve the health of their populations, it is imperative that good quality education is available to all its citizens. Once education standards start to drop, and students fall behind, it is very difficult to make up for it. Public health interventions that compromise education must therefore be implemented with great caution, if at all.

In South Africa, the Reading Panel 2030 report highlighted that 78% of grade 4 learners (students aged 9 turning 10) could not read for meaning. This follows decades of degrading primary school learning facilities, and the severe impact of the COVID-19 lockdown on teaching and learning. During the COVID-19 lockdown, whilst those from wealthier backgrounds at private schools typically had access to online learning, this was rarely the case in the government schools attended by 96% of children. The same panel, comprising 18 experts including the commissioner of the South African Human Rights Commission (SAHRC), predict that it will take 86 years to achieve the desired rate of 95% of grade 4 s being able to read to meaning (Reading Panel 2030, RP 2023). Few South Africans born at the time of writing will live to see that day.

The Whitehall study clearly demonstrates the impact of "employment and working conditions" on health outcomes. In general, the more control employees had over their work, the lower their risk of heart disease—the UK's biggest killer. According to my capacities approach to measuring public health (Chap. 1), having agency at work not only improves health outcomes of that sort, but could itself be a positive health outcome (should that be deemed a "relevant capacity", which given Marmot's findings, it might). To have more agency is to have the capacity to perform a wider variety of tasks, and the capacity to choose which of these one performs. Obviously, employers are generally not in a position to allow their employees to do whatever they want, whenever they want. Certain tasks must be completed. But increased freedom to perform these tasks how and when the employees want is desirable from a public health perspective. Employers are beginning to recognize this, as flexible hours, the ability to work from home, and even a four-day working week are being introduced by many companies worldwide.

Perhaps the biggest constraint on an individual's capacities beyond direct health states (e.g. chronic disabilities) is unemployment. Unemployment can lead to mental health issues, but beyond the depression and anxiety it so often causes (Amiri 2020), are of course the consequences on family income. Without regular work or significant support from the state, people cannot feed themselves or their families, run a household, travel, pay for school or medical supplies, and so on. Unemployment, particularly in developing countries, very often leads to poverty, and little is more incapacitating than poverty. Promoting job growth can thus be seen as a key public health intervention, and as with education, any interventions likely to negatively affect employment should only be taken with extreme caution.

Marmot's fourth recommendation pertains both to reducing poverty, and, following Amartya Sen, to reducing income inequality. There is, as Marmot highlights, more to health inequalities than money, but at lower levels of income, money certainly plays a role.

Following decades of Apartheid, South Africa suffers from both extreme income and wealth inequalities. Reducing wealth inequalities goes beyond reducing unemployment, since the wealth gap is not caused by unemployment alone. According to the Allianz Wealth Report, in South Africa the richest 10% of the population own 70% of net financial assets. Further, wealth distribution can meaningfully be measured by looking at the difference between mean and the median wealth, and in South Africa the mean wealth is 6 times the median, making it the most unequal distribution of wealth measured in the study of 53 countries (the average was 2.5 times the median). The REDI study showed inequality to be even worse, with the top 1% owning 50% of South Africa's wealth, and the top 10% owning 90–95% (Africa Check 2018). Given the country's Apartheid history, it is unsurprising that such a high level of inequality was found.

Whilst South Africa has the highest unemployment rate in the world at 32.9% in the first quarter of 2023 (StatsSA 2023), this is not the sole cause of the wealth gap. Minimum wage in the country is ZAR25.42/hour, currently a little over one British pound Sterling, and just about enough money to buy a litre of petrol or a loaf of bread. The country is characterized by two entirely contrasting ways of living. On the one hand, much of the minority upper-middle-class live in luxury accommodation in secure golf/eco-estates, with their children in high quality private schools, with world class private health care, and many of their homes with generators or solar panels to combat the regular power outages. The vast majority of the country, on the other hand, live either in rural townships, or high population density urban informal settlements.

The majority of dwellings in informal settlements are made of corrugated iron sheets, lack proper sanitation/running water/toilets, and one small property might house as many as 10 people. The public hospitals are chronically overcrowded and under-resourced (e.g., in 2023, newborn babies were discovered in cardboard boxes in the neo-natal intensive care unit at Mahikeng Provincial Hospital, following a shortage of incubators (TimesLive 2023)), and many either have no access to electricity or have dangerous and illegal connections to the power supply—which, as I just mentioned, is at best unreliable.

The primary and secondary school education systems for the poor are in a shocking state. Many have "pit toilets", into which young children can (and do) fall and drown (Al Jazeera 2023), and as discussed earlier in this chapter, the statistics for reading for meaning are dire. The poor endure cholera outbreaks, are more affected by infectious diseases like tuberculosis and HIV (Whiteside 2002), and unsurprisingly were the most severely affected by food insecurity when COVID-19 lockdowns were implemented (Berg et al. 2022). Whilst the official unemployment rates are unacceptably high, most of those working barely earn enough money to put food on the table.

These two lifestyles are so very different, and yet geographically speaking, it is frequently a mere fence or stream that separates the two. On one side of the fence, the children have all the opportunities in the world. On the other, social mobility is little more than a dream. Even the smartest, most driven individual will struggle to make it out of the informal settlement. The poor people of South Africa, like so many places, lack the capacities necessary to escape their current living conditions. To add insult to injury, the luxury lifestyles that others enjoy are in full view. Given that inequality alone gives rise to poor health outcomes for the less well off, and that poverty deprives people of many kinds of opportunity/capacities, the combination of the two experienced by so many South Africans is truly devastating from a public health perspective.

The six policy objectives of the Marmot Review all aim at increasing the capacities of the population as a whole, and those that comprise it. However, as mentioned, this review targeted England, and the needs of developing countries differ to those of the developed world. I will talk more of context-dependent public health interventions and context-dependent public health ethics in Chap. 3 (Evidence Based Public Health), Chaps. 5 and 6 (public health ethics), and Chap. 7 (decolonizing health), but for now it is worth highlighting that the disease burden in the developing world and the Global South is structured differently to that of the developed world/global north. Whereas the leading causes of mortality in England and Wales are cardiovascular disease and dementia/Alzheimers, the leading causes of death in South Africa are tuberculosis and diabetes mellitus (StatsSA 2021). Whereas nearly everyone in the developed world has access to clean water and electricity, the same cannot be said of many countries in the developing world. 6% of South Africans do not have access to clean water—an unacceptably high number—but South Africa is relatively developed. According to a 2020 WHO report, in Niger, Chad, and the Democratic Republic of Congo, 54% of the population lack access to clean water (WHO/UNICEF 2020). Marmot's list would thus require some additions in these contexts. To supplement those six, developing countries would likely need to include, at a minimum:

- Build and maintain infrastructure to provide access to clean running water for all citizens.
- Build and maintain infrastructure to provide access to electricity for all citizens.
- Adequate and affordable transport for all citizens.
- Protection from infectious diseases (vaccine programmes, ARV treatment for HIV, free and easily accessible antibiotic treatment, etc).
- Nutrition education and, where applicable, food supplements (particularly for young children).

The above list is not exhaustive, but since the infrastructure and medical systems of the developed world already meet these requirements, they would not appear on Marmot's UK-orientated list. Suffice to say, access to basic utilities, transport infrastructure, and healthcare for all are necessary conditions of reducing health inequalities and improving population health more generally.

2.4 Munthe's Integrated Multidimensional Model

Munthe attempts to integrate the "new" goals of public health (those of equality and autonomy) with the traditional goal of improving the aggregated health states of the individuals comprising the population. He does this by examining what autonomy amounts to in the public health context, and concluding that the autonomy goal should in fact be combined with the equality goal, such that the associated goal of public health is "*the promotion of equal (and real) opportunities of everyone to be more healthy*[3]" (Munthe 2008, p. 42).

Munthe considers two ways of interpreting autonomy at the population scale, initially by considering the population as a "superindividual" with its own independent autonomy. He concludes that this makes little sense for two reasons: first, that public health descriptively does not view populations in this way. He argues that the traditional interpretation

[3] Munthe's emphasis.

considers the goal of public health to be to improve public health, where this is measured as an aggregate of the health states of those individuals comprising the population, not the health state of the population as a "superindividual".

Whilst it may be true that this is how the traditional interpretation is typically conceived, this is only part of the story. In addition to promoting the health-related capacities of individuals, I suggest that improving the health state of the population as a complex system is precisely what public health should (in part) aim to do. However, whilst measuring the health of populations is possible by appeal to its public-health ratio (its actual capacities relative to those capacities it *could* have), identifying the autonomous choices of a population as a complex system is hard to imagine. Making autonomous choices requires a conscious mind, and whereas some complex systems (sophisticated biological organisms) have such a thing, others do not. Just as a human heart can be healthy, but cannot make autonomous choices, so the same applies to human populations. Respecting autonomy in this context cannot, therefore, mean respecting the autonomy of the superindividual/population as a complex system.

The second interpretation Munthe considers is aggregating the choices/attitudes of the individuals comprising the population, in order to determine the autonomous choice of the population *en masse*. He rejects this approach, too, suggesting that "the degree of measurability required by taking the step to an aggregation of individual autonomy states over a population seems so far removed from what any concept of autonomy allows that avoiding this line of thought seems as the obviously sensible choice" (Munthe 2008, p. 42). Ultimately, attempting to apply autonomy to populations as a whole seems like a category error. The only autonomy in a population lies within the minds of the individuals that make it up (that's not to say that "the will of the people" cannot be represented democratically. In Chap. 6. I suggest that the democratically determined collective will of the people might be important to public health decision-making, at least in some contexts).

Munthe's conclusion, then, is that public health interventions should aim to provide "equal (and real) opportunities for everyone to be more healthy". This integrates the equality and autonomy goals, because whilst "equal opportunities" is inherently egalitarian in nature, the notion of an opportunity admits of allowing individuals to choose not to take said opportunity. When the state introduces the opportunity for all citizens to be vaccinated against some infectious disease, this counts as a new population-level capacity and thus an improvement to the public health ratio (Chap. 1). But the autonomy of the individuals is respected, since nobody is forced to take the vaccine.[4]

Of course, one cannot respect the autonomy of individuals to the extent that anyone can do whatever they want, whenever they want, since this may infringe on the autonomy of others. As Munthe points out, the freedom to smoke in a public area can justifiably be rescinded on the grounds that it infringes on the freedom of others to enjoy a healthy, smoke-free environment. But this caveat—that one retains autonomy unless it interferes with the rights/autonomous choices of others to live a healthy lifestyle—is surely a reasonable one. Indeed, it is a desirable consequence of integrating the equality and autonomy goals; the equality goal provides practical and reasoned constraints on autonomy.

Having integrated the equality and autonomy goals, Munthe moves on to complete his "integrated, multidimensional model" by combining the equality/autonomy goal and the traditional goal of improving public health. Since these goals so often conflict, some means of assessing the complex trade-offs between these competing values is necessary. After considering a number of options, Munthe suggests the following:

- "The more that population health is promoted, the less important it is to promote it further (and vice versa)
- The more that population health is promoted, the more important it is that people may choose not to further promote their health (and vice versa)
- The more that population health is promoted, the more important it is that people have opportunities to further promote their health, which are equally distributed (and vice versa)" (Munthe 2008, p. 45)

[4] I will leave the contentious matter of vaccine mandates and if/when they can be justified to Chap. 7 (public health ethics).

Intuitively it makes sense to suggest that when population health is particularly low, it is considerably more important to focus on improving population health than concerns about equality. However, whilst Munthe assumes that population health is an "aggregate of individual health levels, states, trends etc", the capacities approach I endorse suggests a different way of tackling the problem of goal-integration in the face of (apparently) competing values.

Dissolving the Competing Interests Problem: Invoking the Capacities Approach

The capacities approach to measuring health at the population level takes the health state of the population to be determined by its emergent capacities. The strategy outlined in Chap. 1 admits of evaluative choices in choosing which capacities to prioritize. This allows stakeholders to focus on public health outcomes that promote the "new" goals of equality and autonomy, and leave out capacities that might seem less relevant to the domain of public health—the capacity to put people on the moon, for example.

Whilst the weighting system illustrated in Fig. 2.3 is necessary for Munthe's model, the approach to measuring population health I propose requires no such system. First, the capacities approach draws no distinction between those capacities that improve population health, and those that address inequalities. The traditional goal of improving population health as an aggregate of individual health states (assessed crudely in terms biological dysfunction and/or disvalued physiological/mental states) is abandoned in favour of growing the population's emergent capacities, placing, like Munthe, an emphasis on opportunities over outcomes at the individual level. Second, I contend that, at least in countries like South Africa with high levels of poverty and inequality, the weighting issue Munthe highlights can take care of itself through careful selection of the relevant emergent capacities for population health. Those selected should be those that provide the greatest opportunity for people to improve their individual health.

As discussed in detail in Chap. 1, in the context of individual health states, Sander Werkhoven argues for an unrestrictive dispositional account—the more dispositions the patient has, whatever capacities/dispositions those may be, the healthier they are (Werkhoven 2019). He grants that many pathological conditions confer dispositions on patients (epilepsy confers the disposition to have seizures when certain stimulus conditions are met), but those dispositions are always offset by the many more dispositions the patient loses due to their condition. A similar situation arises in the context of public health. On the one hand, gaining or losing the capacity to access clean water, to avoid food insecurity, or to have access to antiretroviral medications in a region with high HIV prevalence, has implications for thousands of other capacities. On the other, upgrading the healthcare situation of those already in a privileged situation; say, by providing access to gene sequencing for the early detection of risk factors for hereditary diseases, whilst certainly adding to the capacities of that individual, has nowhere near the same impact on the capacities of the population as the kinds of intervention targeting the disadvantaged noted above. In this way, the weighting issue resolves itself, since improving health outcomes for the disadvantaged already has a more positive impact on the capacities of the population (more healthy individuals corresponds to more emergent capacities at the population level), than improving health opportunities or outcomes for the privileged.

Health economics is a sophisticated business, the details of which extend beyond the scope of this book. That said, it is all very well arguing that providing access to clean water for those in poverty has more impact than providing gene sequencing for the rich, but one must consider the costs involved. Building a dam and all the necessary infrastructure to provide clean water is an expensive project, as is providing a reliable power supply to an entire population. Countries that lack that kind of infrastructure, also often lack the resources to provide them—at least not all at once. Similarly, whilst the individual costs of gene sequencing and analysis are high, the overall cost to the fiscus is significantly less than building substantive water or electricity infrastructure. However, I maintain that the public health benefit per dollar spent is typically notably higher where that money is spent on the disadvantaged.

Not all public health interventions are so expensive. Some might be more educational in nature—spending money on health communication or sex-education, highlighting the risks of unprotected sex in regions with a high prevalence of sexually transmitted diseases, for example. Providing free condoms and sanitary pads for disadvantaged teenagers at high school and/or university is a cost effective intervention, where the positive impact on population health can be enormous. The prevention of HIV through condoms will prove significantly cheaper in the long run than providing life-long ARV treatment, and although menstruation is of course not pathologic, its effect on young women's educational experience can (i) be very traumatic if they have no access to the appropriate products, and (ii) have a notable effect on their learning and the many capacities associated with education.

Although it is often the case that academics writing in this space need to be critical of governments, and highlight areas for improvement, it is also worth noting successes. The South African government have placed great emphasis on reproductive health and menstrual hygiene. May 28th is Menstrual Hygiene Day in South Africa. In 2019/2020 the South African minister of finance allocated ZAR157 million to providing free sanitary products to public schools around the country, and NSFAS (the university funding scheme) offered ZAR275 a month for sanitary products for supported students (Government, SA 2019). This initiative has had enormous public health benefits, and can be considered a real victory for women's rights in the country.

2.5 The Goal of Public Health: The Capacities Approach

In this chapter I have applied my approach to measuring health (at both the individual and population level) to various attempts at cashing out the goal of public health, and hinted at what the goal of public health would be under the capacities approach. Let me now be more explicit.

Public health interventions typically aim to improve individual health outcomes. But, as Munthe notes, respect for indiviudal autonomy means that members of the population should, in at least some instances, be able to opt out. The goal of public health should not, therefore, be improving aggregated individual health outcomes, but providing the means through which individuals can improve their health outcomes should they choose to. As a result, the goal of public health should be tied to the emergent capacities of the population (including the services the state are able to provide), as well as the capacities/health of the individuals comprising that population.

I suggest the capacities that make up the public health ratio (Chap. 1) should be chosen by the relevant experts in a consultative process. These can be chosen in such a way as to promote reducing inequalities. Prioritizing access to quality primary and preventative healthcare for all, access to clean water and sanitation for all, electricity for all, quality education for all, and so on, are all possible examples of such capacities. All this should be done with public health ethics in mind. In Chap. 6, through the lens of public health ethics, I examine in more detail which capacities might form the bedrock of this system.

2.6 Conclusion

I began this chapter by examining the traditional interpretation of the goal of public health. This focused on maximizing the aggregate health states of those comprising the population, and excludes any consideration of autonomy or equality/egalitarian values. Whilst Brülde provides a plausible way of making sense of the traditional interpretation through his Moderated HALEs Approach, I reject his account for two central reasons: first, because measuring public health simply as an aggregate of individual health states is misguided, and second, because his approach remains silent on many of what should be considered real public health issues.

Munthe's "Multidimensional, Integrated Approach" integrates the traditional goal of improving public health outcomes, with what he considers to be the competing goals of autonomy and equality. Whilst Munthe's approach is preferable to the traditional goal, I argued in this chapter that the capacities approach to measuring public health deals with the apparent conflicts between health outcomes and autonomy/equality, without the need for any kind of weighting system. When the health of a population is measured by its public health ratio, and appropriate capacities are selected as those deemed relevant to population health, the most effective way of improving the capacities of the population will often be to focus attention on the disadvantaged. This is largely because interventions addressing issues related to poverty and inequality, result in greater improvements to population-level capacities (and indeed aggregated individual capacities) than interventions improving the conditions of the privileged.

"Following the science" alone cannot guide public health policymaking. Only once the goals of public health are clearly defined can science be employed to identify how best to achieve these goals. If, as I suggest, the goal of public health is to promote the capacities relevant to population health, then any interventions that restrict capacities must be carefully weighed up against the capacities they protect. It's worth noting at this point that many of the issues raised are equally relevant to the ethics of public health. After all, the shift from the traditional interpretation to those including egalitarian issues was largely motivated by ethical considerations. In Chaps. 5 and 6, I examine various approaches to public health ethics, and propose a capacities-based, principlist ethical framework.

3

Evidence Based Public Health

3.1 Outline

In this chapter I outline and endorse Evidence-Based Public Health (EBPH), noting that its basic principles have recently (at the time of writing) been largely ignored at important times. And further, that more careful consideration of these principles should lead to better public health outcomes. In order to fully grasp the context, I begin the chapter by looking at Evidence Based Medicine (EBM), the principles and clinical guidelines of which overlap significantly with EBPH (Mercuri and Upshur 2023).[1]

EBM promotes the use of best evidence in clinical decision making, primarily obtained from randomized controlled trials (RCTs) and other large-scale clinical studies. It proposes a hierarchy of evidence (Sackett et al. 1996) on which clinical decisions can (in part) be grounded. EBPH follows a similar approach, with its own hierarchy of evidence tailored to public health policy decisions (Brownson et al. 2009).

[1] This chapter is adapted and significantly developed from previous work published in The Routledge Handbook of the Philosophy of Evidence (Smart 2023a)

B. Smart, *The Philosophy of Public Health*,
https://doi.org/10.1007/978-3-031-98804-2_3

In Sect. 3.2, I discuss the evidence hierarchy proposed by EBM, which ranks different types of evidence based on the "internal validity" of a method, relative to hypotheses regarding efficacy of tested medical interventions (Brownson et al. 2009). In Sects. 3.3 and 3.5, I consider the core tenets of EBPH, largely endorsing them, and highlight some challenges for the movement. I demonstrate that several recent (and poor) important public health decisions paid little attention to some of these tenets—specifically those concerning the importance of context-dependency in policymaking. The lessons learned from these mistakes, I argue, could make a significant difference to public health decision making. In Sect. 3.6, I briefly outline and critique Stegenga's (2018) "Master Argument", which he claims demonstrates that our confidence in hypotheses concerning the effectiveness of medical interventions based on clinical trials should be low. Drawing on Stegenga, I end the chapter by considering the possibility that public health knowledge (that a public health intervention will work) is impossible. However, I tentatively conclude that an externalist approach to knowledge might provide a more positive outlook.

3.2 An Introduction to Evidence Based Medicine

Medicine has long failed to consistently cure common ailments (Porter 2004; Stegenga 2018). In the 1990s, these failures motivated a methodological revolution in clinical practice at McMaster University, giving rise to EBM. Proponents of EBM sought to understand why medicine had such a poor track record, concluding that it was, at least in part, a consequence of the kind(s) of evidence medical practitioners relied on in their clinical decision making.

To resolve this, EBM introduces a hierarchy, organizing various types of evidence into a partially ordered set. This hierarchy ranks methods based on their internal validity concerning tested medical intervention efficacy hypotheses. Several attempts have been made to construct evidence hierarchies, with the Oxford Centre for Evidence-Based Medicine producing a widely recognized table that encapsulates the prevailing sentiment (Phillips et al. 2009) (Table 3.1).

The hierarchy prioritizes randomization, with the apex of the hierarchy devoted to variations on the RCT theme. In an RCT, participants are typically randomly assigned to (at least) two groups: one receiving treatment, and the other receiving a placebo, with (ideally and in principle) neither the participants nor the investigators aware of the allocation until the study's end. This randomization raises the probability that any differences in outcomes between the groups are due to the treatment (Sackett and Rosenberg 1995).

Additional epidemiological evidence can come from observational studies, where investigators do not intervene. In cohort studies (one form of observational study, also called prospective studies), a group (or cohort) is followed, comparing their exposures and outcomes. Conclusions are drawn about the relationships between exposures and outcomes, such as dietary and exercise patterns, cause of death, and disease incidence, as seen in the Framingham Heart Study (Wilson et al. 1987). Cohort studies are powerful, but time-consuming.

In another form of observational study—case-control studies (retrospective studies)—a class of people with disease D (the case group) are compared to a class of people without D (the control group), to assess whether the exposure of interest is more common in the case group. These studies are often conducted in hospital settings, and are relatively

Table 3.1 The EBM hierarchy

Level	Therapy/prevention, aetiology/harm
1a	Systematic review (with homogeneity) of RCTs
1b	Individual RCT (with narrow confidence interval)
1c	All or none
2a	Systematic review (with homogeneity) of cohort studies
2b	Individual cohort study (including low quality RCT; e.g. <80% follow-up)
2c	"Outcomes" research; ecological studies
3a	Systematic review (with homogeneity) of case-control studies
3b	Individual case-control study
4	Case-series (and poor quality cohort and case-control studies)
5	Expert opinion without explicit critical appraisal, or based on physiology, bench research or "first principles"

quick, but can be susceptible to confounding and have limited generalizability (Broadbent 2013).

At the lowest tier on the hierarchy are evidence from laboratory experiments and expert opinions/intuition. EBM challenges the significance of lab results and expert opinions in determining treatment effectiveness, emphasizing that results must translate to real-world outcomes.

EBM offers clinicians evidence-based rules for interpreting literature on disease etiology, prognosis, diagnostics, and treatment, avoiding overreliance on error- and bias-prone intuition. To help medical practitioners apply clinical research to their decision-making, The Evidence-Based Medicine Working Group published "*The Users' Guides to the Medical Literature*" (Guyatt and Drummond 1993).

Somewhat crudely, *The Users' Guide* encourages clinicians to seek the highest available evidence on the hierarchy to minimize biases in decision-making and select the most suitable treatment. The hierarchy allows small quantities of higher forms of evidence to override large quantities of lower forms. For instance, a single high-quality RCT can outweigh multiple observational studies, as seen in the Hormone Replacement Therapy (HRT) trial (Broadbent 2019a, p. 134). EBM does not ignore the role of patients' values in clinical decision-making, but the emphasis is generally on the disease (and clinical trials), rather than the unique qualities of the patient. The system's simplicity makes EBM appealing, but it is not immune to criticism.

Objections to EBM

RCTs, whilst not entirely eliminating bias and confounding, aim to provide an exact quantitative estimate of error probability (Broadbent 2019b, p. 137). As mentioned, in an RCT participants are typically randomized into intervention and control groups, where one group receives the intervention and the other a placebo. Proper randomization should distribute causally relevant factors evenly between the groups, except for the intervention/placebo. This (again, in principle) ensures that any later differences in outcomes can be attributed to the intervention. For example, when testing a new depression drug, randomization ensures a roughly equal number of smokers in both groups, making smoking's impact on depression observable in both.

EBM's unconventional approach to medical practice and its occasionally confrontational stance toward established medical expertise has, however, prompted a number of objections:

Objection (i): The Blinding Objection

RCTs are considered the gold standard of medical evidence due to claims that randomization and blinding eliminate bias and provide accurate insights into the effectiveness of interventions. However, the extent to which RCTs achieve these goals is debatable. RCTs often require a placebo group, and for the trial to provide reliable results, neither investigators nor participants should know if they are receiving (or handing out) the placebo or the treatment during the study. But as Jacob Stegenga highlights, it is often possible for participants to discern which group they are in (Stegenga 2018, p. 155). Many drugs have side effects that the placebos lack, for example. When these side effects are experienced, participants have a good sense of their group assignment.

Objection (ii): The Pill Bias Objection

Some effective interventions are less amenable to blinding than pill-based or injection-based treatments. RCTs, despite their usefulness in assessing the efficacy of pills and intravenous injections, are impractical for assessing the efficacy of surgery, exercise, or mindfulness exercises/meditation (blinding is typically impossible, since participants can easily determine if they've had surgery, exercised, or meditated). Consequently, should evidence-based practitioners insist on placing the greatest emphasis on RCT-supported interventions, many treatment options might be overlooked. This is not because these treatments are ineffective, or even less effective than pharmaceuticals, but rather because conducting RCTs to assess their effectiveness is not feasible. This consequence of the EBM hierarchy has been coined "pill bias" (Broadbent 2019a).

Of course, EBM practitioners do not advocate prescribing only treatments backed by successful RCTs. For instance, exercise is often recommended to overweight patients, even without RCT evidence (other lower forms of evidence that do not require blinding, like case-control studies, can support the associated causal claims). Surgery is frequently considered the most effective (and sometimes the only effective) treatment for numerous pathological conditions. Nonetheless, when treatments with RCT backing are available, EBM prioritizes them over alternatives, inevitably favoring pharmaceutical interventions.

Objection (iii): The Specificity Objection

Specificity presents a similar challenge for EBM to bias. Clinical trials claim to demonstrate the effectiveness of specific interventions on specific populations, but the characteristics of participants in a trial affect its external validity; that is, whether the results of the trial inform the likely success of the treatment on a patient not involved in the trial.

Nancy Cartwright illustrates this external validity issue with two child nutrition projects funded by The World Bank (Cartwright 2012). The first, in Tamil Nadu, India, involved providing nutritional supplements to children and educating mothers about nutrition. The project successfully reduced child malnutrition. As a result of its success, the project was extended to Bangladesh, which faced similar child malnutrition issues. Despite replicating the intervention, the same results were not achieved. In Bangladesh, the supplied food was used as a substitute, not a supplement, apparently because mothers did not hold the same decision-making power regarding child health and nutrition as in Tamil Nadu (this power was handed to the fathers).

Cultural differences between the two regions made the Tamil Nadu study an unreliable indicator of effectiveness in Bangladesh. This problem extends to RCTs and observational studies more broadly. A drug tested in an RCT in the UK or the USA may not have the same effectiveness in Sub-Saharan Africa, due to differing causally relevant contextual conditions.

Furthermore, for safety-reasons, RCTs often exclude groups vulnerable to adverse reactions to medication, e.g., pregnant women, individuals with certain common comorbidities/pre-existing medical conditions like epilepsy or hypertension, and those above or below a certain age (Mulder et al. 2018, p. 5). After a successful clinical trial, however, these excluded groups are often not prohibited from using the drug. Assessing specificity is crucial when evaluating the likely effectiveness of an intervention, and RCTs frequently struggle to accommodate these considerations.

Objection (iv): Reducing Patients to "Statistics"

Related to objection (iii), the nature of the evidence hierarchy has led some critics of EBM to question the applicability of large-scale clinical trials to individual patients. Whilst a particular drug, e.g., a statin, may have a small average effect on reducing heart disease in those with high cholesterol (and thus save hundreds of thousands of lives when prescribed to hundreds of millions of people), there is no way of knowing whether any specific individual will be one of those who benefits from the intervention. Our bodies are all unique, with their own set of dispositions, and individuals can react very differently to the same treatment (Rocca and Anjum 2020). Each patient also has a unique set of values and preferences. This has led to advocates of Patient Centered Care attempting to steer clinicians away from the "cookbook" nature of evidence hierarchies (Mercuri and Upshur 2023), and placing a much larger focus in the clinical decision making process on (1) the unique physiological characteristics of patient, and specifically (2) the individual patient's values and preferences (Epstein and Street 2011).

(v) Publication Bias and Analysis Bias

Sackett (1979) noted 56 types of bias that can influence medical trials. It is beyond the scope of this book to attend to all of them, but it is nonetheless worth mentioning two of the most prominent forms.

Publication Bias

The results of clinical trials are not always positive. Many pharmaceutical interventions turn out to have no beneficial effects for the patient, potentially alongside harmful side effects. A trial may be said to show a significant result when the treatment group had better health outcomes than the control group, and the probability of the null-hypothesis (that this result was down to chance) is less than 5% (a P-value 0.05). However, a trial showing a significant result is far more likely to be published than a trial either showing no significant results, or that the drug causes harm to the patient (Stegenga 2018, p. 160).

This is highly problematic. Suppose 200 trials are conducted on the effectiveness of a drug for hypertension, and suppose *only* positive results get published (this is, granted, an exaggeration). Let us further suppose that the drug is entirely ineffective against hypertension. If the probability of the null hypothesis is (a statistically significant) 5%, then we can expect 10 of these trials to produce positive results through chance alone. But publication bias means that those 10 trials are the ones that get published. The literature now has 10 studies ostensibly demonstrating the effectiveness of the drug with statistical significance, and the 190 trials demonstrating no beneficial effects disappear. This leaves EBM practitioners with only the positive results; wonderful for the profit margins of pharmaceutical companies, but of no help at all to the patients now being prescribed ineffective medication.

Analysis Bias

Given the presence of publication bias, as noted above, and to an extent the sources of research-funding, medical researchers are under pressure to "discover" significant results when they conduct a clinical trial.

Mark Twain once quipped (attributing the remark to British Prime Minister, Benjamin Disraeli) that "There are lies, damned lies and statistics". There are many ways in which one can analyze the data from clinical trials, and often, some methods will produce significant results whilst others do not. This can result in what has become known as "P-hacking", where analysts will try multiple strategies in their data analysis to produce the most convenient results—typically, results showing a pharmaceutical intervention to be effective. Again, suppose that spurious causal relationships will be discovered in 5% of the statistical tests—if an analyst tries 200 different strategies, they are likely to find 10 producing the desirable outcome.[2]

Each of these five objections is reflected in EBPH, and since this is a book on the philosophy of public health, not clinical medicine, I restrict my responses to these objections to the EBPH context.

3.3 An Introduction to Evidence Based Public Health

The application of EBM to public health requires development. Randomization and blinding often pose challenges in public health settings, and public health interventions exhibit significant internal variation, as individuals experience them differently. Whilst a pill is consistent (at least insofar as the pill itself and its consumption during a trial are fairly consistent, even if the patients' reactions to the pill might not be), an advertising campaign aimed at reducing smoking can impact people differently based on factors such as variation in television and social media consumption (Mercuri and Upshur 2023).

EBM, as defined by its founders, requires the explicit and judicious use of the best evidence in clinical settings (Sackett et al. 1996). Following this approach, Jenicek defines EBPH as the "the conscientious, explicit, and judicious use of current best evidence in making decisions about the care of communities and populations in the domain of health protection, disease prevention, health maintenance and improvement (health promotion)" (Jenicek 1997, p. 190). According to Brownson et al. (2018), a consensus exists that decision-making in public health should consider scientific evidence, values, resources, and context.

Despite the known challenges of EBM in clinical settings, applying this approach to public health decision-making is, in my opinion,

[2] See Stegenga (2018) for an excellent discussion of these issues, along with examples.

compelling. Failure to consider scientific evidence can lead to wasteful expenditure on ineffective interventions (I reconsider what should count as suitable evidence in Chap. 7, on decolonizing medicine); failure to acknowledge values and context can lead to the implementation of interventions that, whilst effective elsewhere, fail to have the desired effect in *this* region; and failure to consider the available resources might render some interventions unfeasible. These definitions underscore the importance of having a suitable evidence-base, and of considering the needs, context, and resources of affected communities. In public health crises, adhering to these principles becomes critical, as failing to do so can have devastating consequences.

Brownson, Fielding and Maylahn thus propose three categories of evidence in public health:

- Type 1 evidence defines the causes of diseases and the magnitude, severity, and preventability of risk factors and diseases. It suggests that "something should be done" about a particular disease or risk factor.
- Type 2 evidence describes the relative impact of specific interventions that do or do not improve health, adding "specifically, this should be done".
- Type 3 evidence (of which we have the least) shows how and under which contextual conditions interventions were implemented and how they were received, thus informing "how something should be done". (Brownson et al. 2009)

Epidemiologic studies supply Type 1 and Type 2 evidence, where the EBM movement emphasizes specific Type 2 evidence for clinical decision-making. However, many major public health successes cannot be attributed to RCTs. Identifying the causal link between smoking and lung cancer did involve an RCT, yet this link is well-established. Furthermore, RCTs can be unsuitable when immediate precautionary action is required, such as addressing a pandemic through non-pharmaceutical interventions. RCTs are therefore not ranked above observational studies in the EBPH hierarchy.

Type 3 evidence addresses the specificity concerns of the previous section, focusing on the particular contextual conditions in which an intervention is implemented, and the corresponding outcomes. However, this form of evidence is relatively scarce. This is problematic, since contextual conditions significantly influence intervention effectiveness, as evidenced by the World Bank's Tamil Nadu/Bangladesh child nutrition projects discussed earlier.

At the population level, contextual conditions encompass diet, living arrangements, healthcare access, cultural factors, age, common comorbidities, and so on. Global health crisis recommendations, like pandemic responses, can be ill-advised when they fail to consider population-specific contextual conditions. For example, lockdown policies that might work for some first-world countries, may have different direct and indirect health consequences in third-world countries with younger populations, economic vulnerabilities, and higher population densities (Broadbent et al. 2020). Close consideration of contextual conditions is thus always vital in public health policymaking.

3.4 Evidence in Evidence Based Public Health

EBPH, like EBM, employs an evidence hierarchy. Public health encompasses more evidence types than clinical medicine, where the position each type in the hierarchy occupies depends on its degree of "objectivity". Greater objectivity elevates a form of evidence in the hierarchy, whilst increased subjectivity lowers its rank (Table 3.2).

Like EBM, EBPH places systematic reviews at the hierarchy's pinnacle. As noted above, and unlike its EBM equivalent, it refrains from dictating study preferences (RCTs over observational studies), which could circumvent some issues noted with EBM, especially the pill-bias objection. Nonetheless, the core message remains clear: well-designed studies and systematic reviews should outweigh clinical experience and intuition.

Emphasizing External Validity

The EBM hierarchy, as mentioned, is ordered according to the degree of internal validity those study-types provide. Through the randomization

Table 3.2 *The EBPH Hierarchy* (Adapted from Brownson, Fielding, and Maylahn, 2017)

Level	Evidence
1	Scientific literature in systematic reviews
2	Scientific literature in narrative reviews
3	Scientific literature in one or more journal articles
4	Public health surveillance data
5	Programme/policy evaluations
6	Qualitative data
6a	Community members
6b	Other stakeholders
7	Media/marketing data
8	Word of mouth
9	Personal experience

process, RCTs are considered by many as the gold standard in this regard, since alternative causal explanations for outcome-differences between the intervention and control group are in principle eliminated. Let us assume that an RCT successfully demonstrates the effectiveness of an intervention in a trial. How useful is this to public health policymakers?

Whilst the effectiveness demonstrated in the trial provides good evidence that the same intervention will work under identical circumstances, those circumstances are unlikely to be perfectly replicated in other regions. This is reflected in the Specificity Objection to EBM. Of course, the internal validity of a trial is important, but public health policymakers should typically be equally interested in whether the results of the trial are exportable to the contextual conditions of the population for which the intervention is being considered—the external validity of the trial outcomes.

Unfortunately, the evidence required to ascertain external validity is generally Type 3 evidence, which is often not readily available. In this regard, Brownson et al. note that:

> For public health practitioners, these data on external validity are likely to be as important as information on the internal validity of a particular program or policy. Yet detailed information on external validity is often

> missing in journal articles. Similarly, systematic reviews have difficulty in examining whether factors that may affect external validity (e.g., training and involvement of staff, organizational characteristics) function as important effect modifiers. (Brownson et al. 2018, p. 60)

Given that the data required to establish external validity are frequently missing from epidemiological studies, policymakers must consider the "implementation guides" designed to help stakeholders adapt interventions to their local contextual conditions—but this is far from ideal, and it is advisable that more data be collated prior to implementing a policy that has been shown to work only in different circumstances. Useful data might include: "Key informant interviews… [including] stakeholders at the local level (e.g. program delivery agents, target populations), who have indigenous wisdom about the context for a particular intervention, or the lead investigator or project manager in a research study" (Brownson et al. 2018, p. 60). This form of evidence does appear in the EBPH hierarchy, though it is ranked down at number 6.

In general, a much greater emphasis on external validity in clinical trials is called for. Whilst the very structure of an RCT does not admit of causal conclusions beyond the cohorts involved (or at least not beyond those represented in those cohorts), important contextual considerations could easily be included in the published studies—yet often, they are not. To illustrate this point, Brownson *et al* note:

> Klesges and colleagues reviewed 77 childhood obesity studies to assess the extent to which dimensions of external validity were reported. Importantly, the work of Klesges shows that some key contextual variables (e.g., representativeness of settings, program sustainability) are missing entirely in the peer-reviewed literature on obesity treatment. This finding is likely to apply across most other areas of public health. (Brownson et al. 2018, p. 60)

A change to this trend, with more of a focus on external validity and reporting of the contextual variables required for that, could prove enormously useful to public health policymakers.

3.5 Difficulties for Evidence Based Public Health

EBPH faces a number of challenges—unsurprisingly, some of these correspond closely with those noted above regarding EBM. Mat Mercuri and Ross Upshur highlight three that require specific attention: "methodological constraints (that is, impacts on internal validity), the acute versus chronic nature of the health risk, and equity concerns…" (Mercuri and Upshur 2023).

Methodological Constraints: Blinding, Control Groups, and Context

Whereas a well-designed RCT can provide a reliable estimate of the effect size of e.g., a pharmaceutical intervention, the nature of public health interventions makes this far more difficult. The blinding issue noted with respect to EBM in Sect. 3.2 is commonplace, since with the exception of pharmaceutical-based public health interventions, it will generally be very clear which group one is a part of. One cannot conduct a blinded trial on lockdowns, mask-wearing, hand-washing, or compulsory physical education classes. Similarly, well-designed trials of the kind appearing in the EBM and EBPH hierarchies tend to require a control group, and identifying a suitable control group can give rise to both practical and ethical problems.

During the COVID-19 pandemic we saw different governments implementing very different public health strategies. In the global north, Sweden adopted far less draconian non-pharmaceutical interventions than the norm. Whilst gatherings of more than 50 people were banned in Sweden, and restrictions were put in place on visiting care homes for the elderly, and restaurants and bars were table service only, there were no compulsory lockdowns or curfews in sense we saw across most of Europe. On the face of it, Sweden would thus serve as a reasonably adequate control group for testing the efficacy of lockdown strategies against COVID-19. One might compare the infection and mortality rates of

Sweden with a neighboring country, like Norway, and take the differences to be attributable to the differing interventions.

At the time of writing, Sweden has recorded 2429 deaths/million people, and Norway the significantly lower number of 1024, *prima facie* indicating that lockdowns were effective at curbing the direct health effects of the virus. Unfortunately, though, salient differences in context make this an untenable strategy. The population density of Sweden is 25/km^2 compared with 14.2/km^2 in Norway. The population of Sweden's largest city, Stockholm, is around 1.6 million people (including surrounding urban areas), whereas the population of Norway's largest city, Oslo, is just over one million (Norway 2021). Higher population-density and larger cities provide better conditions for the spread of infectious diseases, putting Sweden at higher risk than Norway from the outset. Of course, there are many causally relevant differences between Sweden and Norway, two Scandanavian countries that are far more similar to one another than, say, Sweden and any country in Sub-Saharan Africa. The more pronounced these differences, the less reasonable it becomes to consider one a control group for the other.

Moreover, different contextual conditions will often suggest the need for different interventions, and this can be the case even within a single country. This leads to a further methodological and practical issue for EBPH, insofar as where policies need to apply to entire populations, the differing contexts of sub-populations might warrant different intervention strategies. Consider South Africa's COVID-19 lockdown as a paradigm example of this:

South Africa initially imposed one of the world's strictest lockdowns, with citizens unable to leave their homes except to receive medical care or buy groceries, and with a curfew from late afternoon. Whilst these rules applied to all those living in South Africa, they affected its citizens very differently. In Chap. 2, I discussed inequality in South Africa, highlighting how the majority of the middle class live in pleasant, uncrowded suburbs, and the (predominantly black) poor majority live in high population density township (shanty town/informal settlement) conditions. The middle class typically have a stable income, most did not lose that income during lockdown (many were able to work from home), and their children mostly attend private schools with the capacity to implement online learning. The country's high levels of inequality led to very different lockdown experiences for different economic groups, and correspondingly different health outcomes. Whereas the middle class experienced no food insecurity and were able to continue to work or receive an education, most children at government schools received no education whatsoever, and the poor (living hand-to-mouth) faced a choice of ignoring the lockdown to earn money for food, or enduring starvation. Unsurprisingly, the statistics suggest they chose the former option. Consider the two graphs, below, showing the COVID-19 caseload for the wealthy suburban regions (Fig. 3.1) and poorer township regions (Figs. 3.2) of South Africa's Western Cape Province.

During the first wave of South Africa's COVID-19 epidemic, the country imposed very strict lockdown conditions. These restrictions were gradually lifted in stages, with stage 5 being the strictest, and stage 1 the least stringent. One can immediately see a contrast between Figs. 3.1 and 3.2 above. In Fig. 3.1, which pertains to the more affluent areas in South Africa's Western Cape Province, one can see that the peak of the second wave (which occurred during less draconian lockdown conditions) was notably higher than that of the first. This arguably indicates (I am not making any stronger claim than that, and acknowledge the lack of

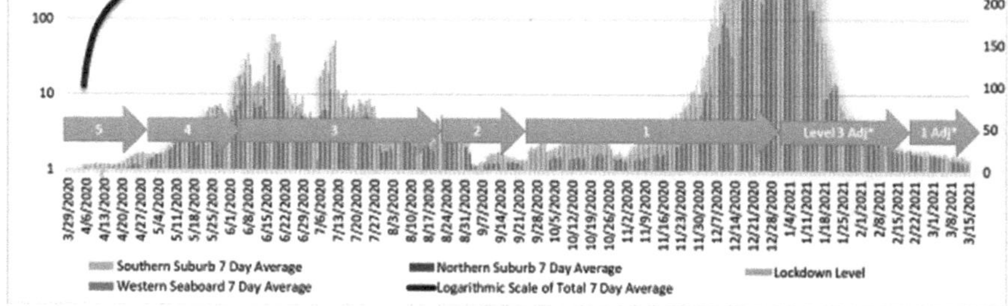

Fig. 3.1 COVID-19 Southern Suburbs, Northern Suburbs, and Western Seaboard caseload (Smart et al. 2021, p. 10)

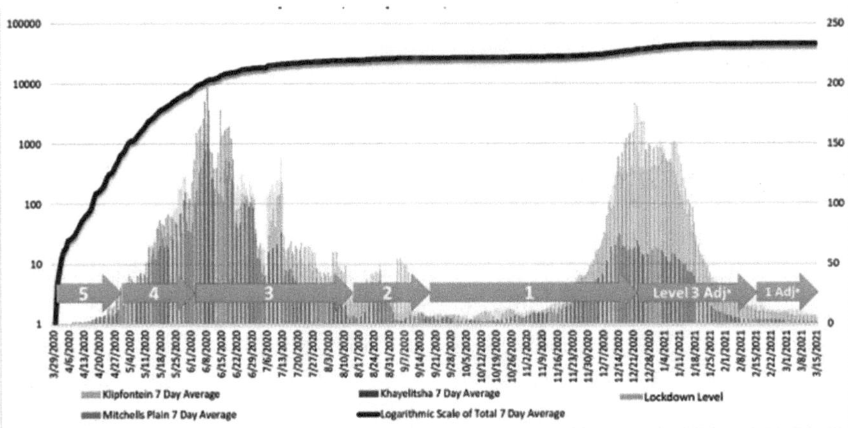

**Adj -Adjusted*

Fig. 3.2 COVID-19 Klipfontein, Khayelitsha, and Mitchells Plain caseload (Smart et al. 2021, p. 10)

scientific rigour, here) that the hard lockdown (level 5) could have had a substantial impact on the spread of COVID-19 among the middle class. This is *prima facie* not the case, however, for the poorer areas of the same province. In Klipfontein, Khayelitsha and Mitchells Plain, where citizens live in the harsh conditions described above, there was no discernable difference between the peaks of the two waves.

Lockdown did not, at least on the face of it, significantly help the poor majority. It did, however, increase food insecurity (Headey et al. 2020), increase unemployment and mental health issues (Posel et al. 2020), and make access to both medical care/preventative medicine (Bulled and Singer 2020) and education far more difficult, if not impossible. I will discuss these issues at greater length in the next section, but suffice to say, the evidence suggests that if lockdown benefitted anyone in South Africa's Western Cape, it benefitted primarily the rich.

So where does this leave public health policymakers? The evidence available could surely have told policymakers that this was a likely outcome. Proper communication with community members, and just a very basic understanding of the living conditions of the poor (paying attention to context), would have allowed policymakers to predict the almost inevitable, and wholly understandable, lack of compliance with the lockdown restrictions.

EBPH stresses the importance of context in public health decision making, acknowledging that one-size-fits-all approaches to public health interventions are rarely ubiquitously effective, and the contexts of the middle class and the poor in South Africa are so very different. But of course, locking down the middle class and applying a Sweden-style approach to those living in townships would have been practically/legislatively impossible, politically extremely unpopular, and arguably not (overall) particularly effective at the national level, given that the middle class make up a relatively small proportion of the total population. Ultimately, public health related legislation (including that imposed during states of emergency) will generally apply universally, and thus governments and other policymakers must look at how best to achieve the goals of public health at the national level.

The Acute Versus the Chronic Nature of the Health Risk

Mercuri and Upshur (2023) note that public health policymakers are sometimes faced with a dilemma: act now in the absence of the evidence one would normally require for whatever interventions are proposed, or wait for the appropriate evidence to materialize, and risk the effects of failing to act in good time. When a public health emergency strikes, such as a dangerous epidemic, the population can face an immediate and severe health risk. The 2020 COVID-19 pandemic can be considered a good example of this. In these instances, those working in public health often appeal to "the precautionary principle".

The precautionary principle enables policymakers to take action when (1) the effects of an intervention are scientifically uncertain, and (2) the risks associated with failing to act are (or at least could be) particularly high (Goldstein 2001). In early 2020, when COVID-19 became a global pandemic, there was enormous uncertainty at many levels. This is reflected in the inaccurate predictions offered by those modelling the projected course of the epidemic. The UK relied heavily on the Imperial

College London Model when developing its response to the pandemic, but for almost all countries modelled by this group, considerably more deaths were predicted than materialized (Magness 2021). Neil Ferguson's team at Imperial College projected 66,393 deaths after 1 year in Sweden should they take an "unmitigated" approach, and 30,434 deaths should they lock down. Sweden recorded 13,396 deaths from COVID-19 in that period—an overestimate of 392%. The same consortium projected 510,000 deaths in the UK in the unmitigated scenario. The UK implemented lockdown strategies based on these projections. In the face of half a million potential deaths, it seems natural to think that doing something is better than doing nothing, even if we don't quite know how effective the interventions will be, and understand that it will have significant effects on the economy and education.

Despite the inaccuracies of the model, Adam Biggs and Lanny Littlejohn, in a commentary published in *The Lancet*, state that "initial projections were commendable efforts that brought about public action despite more than 2 million deaths in the USA and more than 500,000 deaths in the UK being a significant overestimation" (Biggs and Littlejohn 2021). I take this to be a particularly interesting comment, because it makes no reference to the model's accuracy, other than to say it was a "significant overestimate" (a negative remark). Ferguson's work is not being praised, it seems, for its quality or accuracy, but for its ability to motivate politicians to act during a public health emergency. The overestimated figures pushed policymakers to invoke the precautionary principle, and without knowing what the impact of either the virus or the non-pharmaceutical interventions would be, to impose nationwide lockdowns.

Of course, applications of the precautionary principle are not without their controversy. In this instance, given the impact of lockdown on the economy, on education, on areas of healthcare unrelated to COVID-19, and many other aspects of daily life (all affecting our capacities as a population), I am personally not convinced that providing policymakers with inaccurate figures can be considered particularly commendable, even if (1) the lockdowns were an effective intervention, and (2) providing more accurate figures a borderline impossible task.

It is of course quite possible that even with more accurate figures, the same decisions would have been made. More than 200,000 people died of COVID-19 in the UK, even with the non-pharmaceutical interventions in place, and it is extremely difficult to say what that number would be in the counterfactual unmitigated scenario. I of course acknowledge the benefit of hindsight, and that modelling the mortality rates of a new infectious disease is exceptionally difficult, but despite all of this, if the benchmark for "commendable" modeling is to motivate policymakers, then modelers will be tempted to systematically and intentionally use parameters that tend to overestimate the impact of diseases—this is surely an undesirable state of affairs.

Ultimately, policymakers must weigh up the short-term benefits of an intervention like lockdown, with the longer-term adverse consequences. Whilst the global economy, at least to a large extent, recovered relatively quickly (Jiang et al. 2022), many people lost their jobs during the pandemic due to the non-pharmaceutical interventions policymakers implemented, and the global inflationary consequences of economic interventions were substantial. In South Africa, testing for HIV and tuberculosis was significantly reduced (Hogan et al. 2020), and routine tests for cancer and other chronic diseases all but stopped due to both the cancellation of routine appointments and surgical procedures in public hospitals, and transportation difficulties during lockdown conditions. Early detection for all these diseases is crucial if they are to be successfully treated. Amputations due to diabetes increased (Caruso et al. 2020), mental health issues such as depression and anxiety increased, and education for the disadvantaged stopped—worsening the already dire state of education in the country. In short, extreme public health interventions involve substantial trade-offs, and it is vitally important that high quality cost-benefit analyses be conducted before acting. Whilst acting quickly is necessary if complete suppression of the infection is to be achieved, this should not be implemented without due consideration of both the short- and long-term consequences, whatever the circumstances.

Equity Considerations and Evidence Based Public Health

In Chap. 2., The Goals of Public Health, I placed some emphasis on how the capacities approach to measuring public health tends to promote a focus on disadvantaged groups. But were EBPH to focus predominantly on promoting those interventions that perform best in clinical trials (where possible), equity considerations might be largely ignored. In the context of EBM, Mercuri and Upshur note that:

> Equity issues are not the target of measurement in clinical trials, where the purpose is to determine an unbiased estimate of effect. Whilst the GRADE framework acknowledges other considerations in making clinical recommendations…, clinical recommendations are highly sensitive to the quality of evidence of the effect estimate (Mercuri and Upshur 2023, p. 151).

Were the EBM hierarchy applied in the public health context, the effect of pill bias would be to promote the distribution of pharmaceutical interventions, which can be difficult for those living in poverty to obtain, and might be far less effective public health interventions than e.g., improving water and sanitation infrastructure, education programmes regarding infectious diseases, nutrition programmes, and so on. Fortunately, EBPH places less of an emphasis on randomized controlled trials than EBM, with the top three evidence-types in the hierarchy being: scientific literature in systematic reviews; scientific literature in narrative reviews; and scientific literature in one or more journals. Moreover, the hierarchy includes public health surveillance data and qualitative data from community members and other stakeholders. This information is fundamentally important to making equitable public health decisions, since it will inform policymakers as to the most urgent needs of the community, and as to what public health interventions are likely to be best received by the community. Any public health intervention, from vaccines to nutrition programmes, will succeed only with the buy-in of the community, so the importance of this cannot be overstated.

EBPH has great potential to promote health equity on an international scale. Whilst health inequality is of course a problem in the global south, the global north is not immune to the problem. In a paper identifying inequality trends in the US, Singh et al. found that

> Black infants and children in poor, rural communities had nearly three times higher mortality rate compared to those in affluent, rural areas. Racial/ethnic, socioeconomic, and geographic disparities were particularly marked in mortality and/or morbidity from cardiovascular disease, cancer, diabetes, COPD, HIV/AIDS, homicide, psychological distress, hypertension, smoking, obesity, and access to quality health care. (Singh et al. 2017)

In response to this, some have advocated the use of "Global Learning", where policymakers in high-income countries learn from low-income countries, implementing low-cost and highly effective public health interventions that have succeeded in the developing world (Ogbolu et al. 2022). These strategies tend to focus on the social determinants of health, taking an evidence-based approach. The strategy is endorsed by the WHO, which in a 2008 report promoted "generating and disseminating social determinants of health knowledge", with the following definition:

> *Generating and disseminating social determinants of health knowledge*: Ensure research funding is allocated to social determinants of health work; support the global health observatory and multilateral, national, and local cross-sectoral working through development and testing of social determinants of health indicators and intervention impact evaluation; establish and expand virtual networks and clearing houses organized on the principles of open access, managed to enhance accessibility from sites in all high-, middle-, and low-income settings;… (WHO Commission on Social Determinants of Health 2008)

The mention of the "development and testing of social determinants of health indicators and intervention impact evaluation", and of open access to this data, highlights the importance the WHO attributes to evidence-based interventions.

3.6 Evidence for Public Health Knowledge

In an ideal world, public health policymakers would *know* that their interventions will be effective (and precisely how effective) in advance, alongside their less desirable consequences. This knowledge would (somewhat trivially) be invaluable for policymakers, who (should) rely predominantly on evidence-forms in the EBPH hierarchy to form those beliefs. However, in *Medical Nihilism* Jacob Stegenga argues that our confidence in the effectiveness of a medical intervention should be low, despite all the evidence provided by clinical trials (Stegenga 2018). This brings into question the very existence of medical/public health knowledge (knowledge that our medical/public health interventions will improve health outcomes). If our confidence in the effectiveness of medical interventions should be low, does medical/public health knowledge exist at all, and if so, under what circumstances?

In this section, I provide an introduction to this debate, ultimately suggesting that externalists about justification will likely have a better claim to public health knowledge than internalists. A comprehensive discussion with fully justified conclusions would likely require an entire book, so I invite others to extrapolate on these ideas.

I start, again, by referring to the (more comprehensive) philosophy of medicine literature. In part because some of our most effective public health interventions (certain vaccine programmes, for example) would be susceptible to the very same objections.

In order to challenge the rationality of our trust in medical interventions, Stegenga presents what he calls the "Master Argument". This draws on Bayes' Theorem, according to which our confidence in a hypothesis (P(H|E)) is given by P(E|H)P(H)/P(E), where (in this context) H is the hypothesis that a medical intervention is effective, and E is the evidence supporting that intervention.

Stegenga argues first that, given the historic failures of medical interventions (see Broadbent 2019b), we should assume a low prior for H, P(H). Second, given various factors commonplace in medical research such as the publication and analysis bias discussed above, P(E) is high;

that is, we should consider it likely that the evidence provided by clinical trials supports the hypothesis. Third, he argues that P(E|H) should be low:

> If E is evidence that the intervention is relatively ineffective (say, the effect size is small), the probability of observing such evidence conditional on the truth of the hypothesis, P(E|H), is low. This is another way of saying that if the intervention were effective, we would expect to get evidence (from a trial, say) that the intervention is in fact effective. Small absolute effect sizes are widespread in medicine. Smaller effect sizes entail lower likelihood of effectiveness hypotheses. (Stegenga 2018, p. 176)

If P(E) is high, and both P(E|H) and P(H) are low, then, he suggests, necessarily P(H|E) is low; that is, we should have little faith in hypotheses concerning the effectiveness of medical interventions based on the results of clinical trials. If Stegenga is right, one should be sceptical of the results of clinical trials, and acknowledge that even the "gold-standard" evidence endorsed by EBM cannot endow us with medical knowledge (and *a fortiori,* public health knowledge that depends on medical knowledge).

Stegenga's argument has been criticized on the grounds of lack of precision in the terms "low" and "high", with no quantitative values assigned to the prior, P(H), or indeed the other variables. As Jon Fuller notes, "if by 'low' probability we mean 0.5 and by 'high' probability we mean 0.25, then plugging in these numbers into Bayes' Rule we get a p(H|E) of 1.0, which does not meet our definition of 'low'" (Fuller 2020, p. 2). Since "low" applies to P(H) and P(E|H), and "high" to P(E), it is not inconsistent to suggest 0.25 is high and 0.5 low—a 25% rate of bias among researchers might well be deemed high, and a prior of 0.5 for a drug that has undergone years of intensive research and development might well be deemed low. This critique highlights the problem (and importance) of quantifying these values. Stegenga primarily justifies attributing low and high values by appeal to historical information and concerns regarding various forms of bias, but establishing warranted quantitative values requires much further work, without which it is difficult to assess the validity of the Master Argument (Fuller 2020).

In the absence of this data, one might remain somewhat sceptical of Stegenga's conclusions. Nonetheless, Stegenga's insights regarding the various biases in medical research, the failure of medicine to provide "magic bullet" cures for so many diseases, and indeed the harm that medicine has caused patients throughout its history, might equally warrant a sceptical approach to mainstream medicine, and in turn to (at least certain aspects of) public health. Do we know whether e.g., a vaccine will work well once widely used, or even whether it is likely to work? Can we even know? I tentatively suggest here that whether medical knowledge (and correspondingly, relevant public health knowledge) is obtainable, at least in part depends on one's philosophical inclinations regarding knowledge itself.

Crudely speaking, epistemologists stand in one of two camps: the externalists and the internalists. What distinguishes knowledge from (mere) true belief is the "warrant" one has for that belief. Externalists and internalists differ in what they consider to be the appropriate warrant. For the internalist, this warrant derives from our internal cognitive perspective—it is accessible through introspection and reflection. For the externalist, the warrant distinguishing true belief from knowledge must come from some source external to one's cognitive perspective. Externalism about knowledge comes in a variety of forms (see "Reliabilism" (Armstrong 1973) and "The Causal Theory of Knowing" (Goldman 1967)), but for all forms of externalism, the knower will not be able to access through introspection the warrant that transforms their true beliefs into knowledge.

Most internalists adopt either the "KK Principle" or the "JK Principle". These state that "for an agent to know that P, the agent must know that they know that P", and that "for an agent to know that P, they must know their justification for their knowledge that P", respectively. More generally, they must know that their belief is warranted through introspection. It's hard to see how the internalist could claim that either the KK or JK principles are satisfied when it comes to beliefs about effectiveness derived from clinical trials. Whilst an RCT provides evidence *that* some intervention is effective, it does not tell you *why* it is effective. For the internalist, I contend, understanding the mechanisms would be key.

The externalist, on the other hand, can be less pessimistic in this regard. Let us consider the two forms of externalism noted above: reliabilism and the causal theory of knowing. It is beyond the scope of this book to do a deep dive into the intricacies of each view and their variations, and Goldman's refined causal theory of knowing (Goldman 1975) is itself a form of reliablilism. But a superficial overview will suffice for my purposes.

Crudely, the reliabilist takes the warrant distinguishing mere true beliefs from knowledge to derive from the source of the belief: a true belief is knowledge if it is obtained from a reliable process (Ramsey 1931). Reliabilist theories have since been developed by Robert Nozick, who suggests that S knows that P if (1) if *P* were not true, then *S* would not believe that *P*, and (2) if *P* were true, *S* would believe that *P* (Nozick 1981); Tim Williamson, who claims that S knows that P if "if *S* believes that *P*, then *P* would not easily have been false" (Williamson 2000), and many others. For the reliabilist, then, the key factor in determining whether a belief could count as knowledge is the reliability of the source of that belief.

We saw in the previous section how Stegenga questions the reliability of clinical trials, going so far as to suggest that our confidence in the results of clinical trials demonstrating the effectiveness of pharmaceutical interventions should generally be low. If Stegenga is right, then clinical trials cannot provide knowledge—they are not reliable. Whether clinical trials are a reliable indicator of effectiveness is not, however, a mind-dependent fact. Medical and public health interventions either work or they do not, and the reliability of clinical trials can only be determined over time, as we see whether trials demonstrating statistically significant (positive) results translate to positive health outcomes in populations.

Regardless of how reliable those processes currently are, more medical and public health knowledge can be obtained by improving the reliability of the processes generating beliefs in the effectiveness of medical/public health interventions. This requires eliminating, to whatever extent is possible, the biases discussed in the previous section (along with the other 54 noted by Sackett!), ensuring randomization is properly applied where appropriate to reduce the impact of confounders, and disincentivizing P-hacking. In public health, it requires that far more attention be paid to factors affecting the external validity of trials, including a greater emphasis on the collation of Type 3 evidence (Brownson et al. 2009). In short, even if the evidence comprising the EBM and EBPH hierarchies does not currently provide sufficiently reliable evidence to endow medical practitioners and public health policymakers with medical/public health knowledge, refinement of the processes giving rise to this evidence could in principle lead us in that direction.

For example, according to the Causal Theory of Knowing, "S knows that P if and only if the fact P is causally connected in an "appropriate" way with S's believing P" (Goldman 1967, p. 364). If a trial has been conducted in bad faith with intentional P-hacking, or without due consideration of confounding factors, then the statistically significant results of the trial will not be causally connected in "an appropriate way" with the effectiveness of the drug—regardless of whether that drug is effective. But many trials are well-designed, conducted in good faith, and using the most appropriate forms of randomization to eliminate the effect of confounders. Where the trials are well-designed, the analysts pay close attention to the potential effects of bias, and the intervention is indeed effective, then a statistically significant result surely can be causally connected to the effectiveness of the intervention in a way that would satisfy Goldman's criteria—this opens the door to medical/public health knowledge.

Unfortunately, medical practitioners and public health policymakers are not always in a position to easily distinguish between well-designed trials, and those conducted in bad faith. Furthermore, the dearth of type-3 evidence makes external validity a real issue. Clinicians will thus typically not know whether their beliefs about the likely effectiveness of an intervention are appropriately warranted. However, neither the KK nor JK principles are endorsed by externalists, so this does not prevent them from knowing that an intervention is effective. So long as their beliefs are tied to the facts in an appropriate way, knowledge remains possible.

A greater focus on Type 3 evidence (greater understanding of contextual conditions), and more focus on eliminating the various biases highlighted by Sackett, will improve the ratio of positive clinical trials that translate into effective interventions in the field, to those that ultimately prove ineffective. In turn, this should result in more public health knowledge (for the externalist). I acknowledge that the arguments presented here may not be fully convincing, and require further development. However, regardless of whether I'm right in that the externalist might have a greater claim to public health knowledge than the internalist, I hope this section serves to provide motivation for improving the reliability of our evidential standards.

3.7 Conclusions

The EBM hierarchy is structured according to the degrees of internal validity of each type of evidence. In public health, whilst internal validity of course remains important, the wide variety of contextual conditions in which different populations live make the transportability of results to other contexts absolutely vital. The EBPH hierarchy correspondingly differs from the EBM hierarchy—it is structured according to the objectivity/subjectivity of the evidence-types, with less of an emphasis on randomization (observational studies are not ranked higher than RCTs). Importantly, the EBPH hierarchy includes qualitative data from community members and other stakeholders. With this information, policymakers can draw on indigenous knowledge about the local community and their contextual/cultural conditions, and use this to determine how likely the proposed intervention is to work in that area and/or what modifications need to be made to tailor it to that community. Failure to do this can have unfortunate consequences, as Cartwright demonstrated using the Tamil Nadu/Bangladesh case study.

Whilst the EBPH hierarchy generally advocates implementing interventions based on literature highlighting the effectiveness of interventions, and much of this literature pays little attention to equity concerns, public health policymakers can use their discretion in implementing those policies that best reflect their overall goals. Given that, as I have argued in previous chapters, public health is best improved by focusing on building population-level capacities, policymakers (particularly in the developing world) should shift their focus to evidence-based interventions that best provide opportunities for the vulnerable and disadvantaged to improve and sustain their health. Furthermore, to avoid policy mistakes caused by implementing inappropriate context-specific interventions, more of an emphasis should be placed on both gathering and utilizing Brownson et al.'s Type 3 evidence in public health.

4

The Metaphysics of Public Health

4.1 Outline

In this chapter, I consider several metaphysical questions in the philosophy of public health. These can be split into two broad categories, though often the demarcation in the literature between the two is subtle or entirely missing. On the one hand, there are ontological questions. These concern the *nature* of the entities or processes involved. On the other, there are questions pertaining largely to conceptual analysis; that is, what particular concepts mean, given the context. Both are important, and both will be addressed.

Since the health of individuals comprising a population plays such a key role in population health, in Sect. 4.2. I start with models of disease causation. These have both conceptual and ontological components. Given the direct impact of disease on public health, I examine the literature on disease-etiology, presenting and evaluating a both the monocausal (Koch 1884) and multifactorial (Rothman 2012) schools of thought. This mainly pertains to the project in conceptual analysis, but there are ontological implications. I end the section with the dispositional model

B. Smart, *The Philosophy of Public Health*,
https://doi.org/10.1007/978-3-031-98804-2_4

of disease etiology for diseases in individuals, and in Sect. 4.3. expand this model to the population-scale.

In Sect. 4.4. I move on to the ontology of epidemics. At the time of writing, the philosophical literature on this topic is particularly sparse. Searching for a prescriptive account of epidemics—that is, how those working in public health *should* identify epidemics, rather than how they do—I have argued elsewhere that epidemic-status, like health-status, is an emergent property of a complex system (Smart and Combrink 2022). We argue in favour of a value-dependent realist account of epidemics. Here, I develop those ideas, putting them in the context of the capacities approach to measuring the health of populations proposed in Chap. 1.

4.2 The Metaphysics of Disease Etiology

Disease Etiology

In this section I first consider the traditional two-stage model of disease etiology, comprising "illness causation" and "pathomechanism" (MacMahon and Pugh 1970). Illness causation refers to the causal processes leading from a state of health in the patient, to the initial somatic response. For an infectious disease such as Tuberculosis (TB), this would involve the patient's exposure to the pathogen (in the case of TB, *Myobacterium tuberculosis*), perhaps in addition to other causally relevant factors.

Pathomechanism occurs subsequent to illness causation. These are the causal processes within the body leading from the initial exposure (in the case of transmissible diseases) to the primary symptoms characterizing the disease. Many infectious diseases have an incubation period, during which the patient is asymptomatic. But whilst asymptomatic, pathomechanisms are underway that will eventually result in the standard manifestation of disease itself (Dammann and Smart 2019).

Let us assume that the goal of medicine is to return patients with diseases to a state of health. It often cannot achieve this goal, but that is arguably the ideal. Whilst medicine is predominantly concerned with cure (whether a return to complete health, or merely alleviation of symptoms), public health is predominantly concerned with prevention. The two-stage model highlights two possible intervention strategies: to intervene prior to the initial somatic responses, through interference with illness causation, or intervention whilst the pathomechanisms are already underway. However, in the context of public health, this omits an important part of disease etiology, specifically in cases of infectious diseases.

Merav Edout[1] has suggested a third aspect should be added to this model of disease etiology: "Pathogen origination". These, as the name suggests, are the causal processes that lead to new pathogens. COVID-19 is caused by the virus Sars-Cov-2. There are a number of theories concerning the origination of Sars-Cov-2, ranging from the interaction of multiple viruses from more than one infected species at a wet market in Wuhan, to more sinister theories involving leaks from a laboratory where the virus had been intentionally created (Bloom et al. 2021). Whatever the process that led to the first instance of the Sars-Cov-2 virus, that was the "pathogen origination" for every instance of COVID-19.

A public health intervention such as banning wet markets to curtail the development of new zoonotic diseases could well have prevented the largest pandemic (at least in terms of cases) in nearly a hundred years. Public health must therefore not only be cognizant of illness causation, but also of pathogen origination.

Not all diseases fit this model. In the twenty-first century, the dominant causes of global mortality are not infectious diseases, but chronic diseases such as diabetes and cardiovascular disease (Beaglehole and Horton 2010). However, the three-stage model becomes increasingly important to recognize as the pace of zoonotic disease emergence accelerates, becoming a rising threat to public health.

Now that I have established three key (causal) stages leading to the onset of clinical disease, I move on to the metaphysics of disease etiology. Much of the literature on this topic is a debate between monocausal theories of disease, and multifactorial accounts. This is an exercise in conceptual analysis. It is not concerned with the nature of the properties or processes involved, but rather identifying what counts as causes of

---

[1] Paper in preparation.

disease. In the next section I evaluate various views in the literature, before moving on to the ontological aspects of these causal questions.

Monocausal or Multifactorial Accounts of Disease Etiology?

Whilst more recent proponents of multifactorial accounts often present their views as a response to the monocausal model, multifactorial accounts in fact predate the monocausal account by millennia (Ross 2018). Proponents of monocausal accounts consider diseases to be caused by a single causal factor. This single causal factor is often also deemed to play a role in the identification or classification of the disease itself (Smart 2014). In the context of the history of medicine, monocausal accounts are a relatively recent development, deriving in large part from the discoveries of Robert Koch (1884).

Koch discovered that all livestock suffering from anthrax had the same rod-shaped bacteria in their blood; further, that when healthy livestock are inoculated with these bacteria, they too start showing the symptoms of anthrax. Additional research uncovered similar findings with cholera, diphtheria, and tuberculosis: a single pathogen for a single pathological condition. Monocausal theories assume this trend generalizes for all diseases.

Multifactorial accounts reject the monocausal view, suggesting that diseases have multiple causes. When a patient manifests the symptoms of the common cold, it's not only caused by exposure to the pathogen, but also the state of the patient's immune system, and perhaps many other causally relevant factors. Bearing in mind the goal of identifying how medicine and public health (descriptively) identify the causes of disease, in this section I briefly explore the history of these views, present versions of them in more detail, and conclude in favour of Ross's (2018) doctrine of specific etiology. Although Ross rejects the monocausal model simpliciter, her account respects the underlying interventionist principles.

Multifactorial Models

Prior to Koch's discoveries, cholera, now known to be caused by the bacteria *Vibrio cholerae,* was "attributed to a lack of exercise, excessive alcohol consumption, a lack of religious belief, noxious air, bacterial infection, mental exhaustion, and a lack of nourishing food" (Ross 2018, p. 4). These causes were not all viewed as necessary conditions, but nonetheless the disease was thought to be caused by a combination of factors.

Some philosophers, speaking of causation more generally, have suggested that absences can be considered causes. Mackie (1974) argues that causes are insufficient but non-redundant parts of unnecessary but sufficient conditions (*inus* conditions). He includes absences in his analysis. The cause of a child contracting measles is thus not only her exposure to the virus *Rubeola*, but also their failure to be vaccinated against the disease. Ken Rothman captures this idea in the epidemiology literature in his 'Sufficient Cause' model of disease. He represents this idea with causal pies comprising slices, where each slice of the pie represents a causally relevant factor/*inus* condition (Rothman 2012). A complete pie results in disease, but should none of the 'sufficient causes'/pies be complete, the disease will not manifest.

Figure 4.1 above represents the sufficient causes/pies for some disease P to manifest in a patient. The letters A, B, C, D, E, and F represent what Mackie terms *inus* conditions. They can either be a positive contribution, such as exposure to a pathogen, or an absence, such as the failure to be

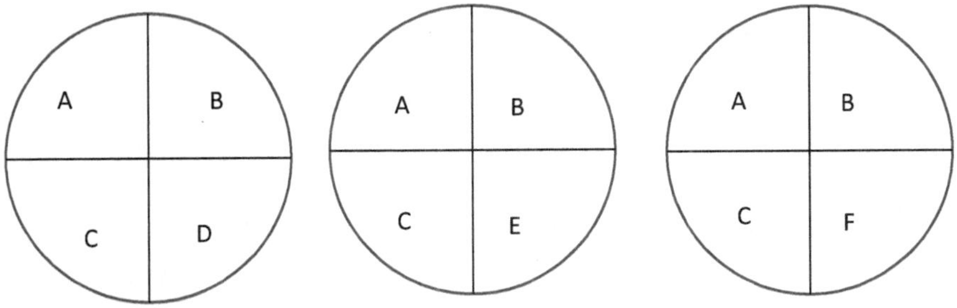

Fig. 4.1 Rothman's sufficient cause model

vaccinated. According to this model, should all the conditions be satisfied in any one of these pies, then the disease necessarily manifests. Since A, B, and C appear in all the sufficient causes, these are necessary conditions for the onset of P. However, A, B, and C are together insufficient. One of conditions D, E or F must also be satisfied, but none of these are necessary conditions for P, since they do not appear in all the sufficient causes.

If we assume absences can be considered *inus* conditions, it is possible for any given sufficient cause to comprise an infinite number of slices. This is not, however, inherently problematic for the model.

I now consider three questions arising from Rothman's sufficient cause model of disease etiology. First, whether it accurately reflects the nature of disease causation (an ontological question, which I expand on later). Second, how public health policy can be shaped by such models (once the *inus* conditions are given determinate referents). And finally, whether Rothman's model reflects how medicine and public health identify causes (the key question from the conceptual analysis perspective).

For Rothman's model to accurately reflect the nature of disease etiology, disease causation must be deterministic; that is, given all the *inus* conditions within any sufficient cause are met, the disease must manifest. There are two issues at hand, here: the metaphysical and the epistemic. From the epistemic perspective, it's incredibly difficult, if not impossible to identify the sufficient causes for at least some diseases. As mentioned, the number of *inus* conditions is potentially infinite, making it literally impossible to specify them all. Further, even were the number of *inus* conditions finite in number, there will always be epistemic uncertainty regarding the completeness of the sufficient causes.

Suppose we believe ABCD above is the accurate sufficient cause for P. Should all the conditions be met, and P fail to obtain, we discover that ABCD is not a sufficient cause after all. However, we do not know whether the sufficient cause model is accurate, and we are simply missing *inus* conditions in our sufficient cause, or whether the sufficient cause model is flawed on the grounds of disease etiology being an indeterministic process. From the epistemic perspective, then, we must take sufficient causes with determinate variables with an appropriate degree of scepticism.

From the metaphysical perspective, the sufficient cause model might well reflect the nature of disease causation—but again, it will only do so if disease etiology is a deterministic process. The sufficient cause model does not allow for all the *inus* conditions comprising a sufficient cause to be met, and the disease to fail to manifest. It is beyond the scope of this book to argue for or against determinism, and there is no consensus on whether we live in deterministic or chancy world. So I can conclude only that whilst there is no way of knowing whether the sufficient cause model accurately reflects the metaphysics of disease etiology, it is possible.

The Sufficient Cause Model Shaping Public Health Policy

Both medicine and public health are disciplines interested in affecting change. They look to interfere with existing states of affairs in order to improve health outcomes for individuals and/or populations. This basic idea forms the basis of the interventionist accounts of disease etiology to be discussed, shortly, but it is also worth noting as we consider how health researchers and policymakers could use Rothman's pies.

In the example above, all three sufficient causes for disease P all include *inus* conditions A, B, and C. Those three conditions are together insufficient for P, but given *ex hypothesi* the three sufficient causes are the only sufficient causes for P, conditions A, B and C are all individually necessary for P. Conditions D, E and F are not, since none of them appear in all three sufficient causes.

A rational strategy for medical and public health interventions is to identify those manipulable *inus* conditions that appear in every sufficient cause. Not all the necessary conditions will be manipulable (for instance, the presence of oxygen is necessary for contracting TB, but it is not manipulable without killing the patient), but hopefully at least some will be. The absence of an effective vaccine, for example, will be an *inus* condition for every transmissible disease. It's no surprise, then, that developing effective vaccines is (or at least should be) given such high priority when dealing with infectious diseases.

Does the Sufficient Cause Model Reflect how Medicine and Public Health Identify Causes?

The presence of oxygen is necessary for any patient to contract any disease. Without oxygen the patient dies. The presence of oxygen must therefore be an *inus* condition in every sufficient cause. Unsurprisingly, when one searches for the causes of disease, the presence of oxygen is never mentioned. It's both trivial, and irrelevant. It's trivial because a patient can't contract a disease if they're dead, and it's irrelevant because medicine and public health are concerned only with conditions that are usefully manipulable. Removing oxygen from the air a patient breathes is neither a viable preventative intervention nor a viable treatment. In short, whilst the sufficient cause model might well accurately reflect the metaphysics of causation, it certainly does not reflect how medicine and public health identify the causes of disease. Theirs is a far more selective approach.

The Monocausal Model

Following his anthrax discovery in the late nineteenth century, Koch developed a set of criteria to establish definitive causal relationships between pathogens and diseases. The criteria emphasize identifying a single microbial cause for a specific disease. Koch's postulates are as follows:

1. The microorganism must be found in abundance in all organisms suffering from the disease but should not be found in healthy organisms.
2. The microorganism must be isolated from a diseased organism and grown in pure culture.
3. Inoculation of a healthy individual with the cultured microorganism must recapitulate the disease.
4. The microorganism must be re-isolated from the inoculated, diseased individual and matched to the original microorganism. (Koch 1884)

These criteria are clearly insufficient, even for infectious diseases. As early as 1937, Thomas Rivers highlighted how they did not apply to viral infections (Rivers 1937), since viruses cannot be cultivated on lifeless media. However, the impact of Koch's work on communicable diseases was, and continues to be, enormous. Viewing disease etiology in this way enabled the development of effective and targeted interventions. Not because the postulates accurately reflect disease etiology—they clearly do not—but due to the shift from vague multifactorial approaches to disease etiology, to what Ross (2018) has coined a "doctrine of specific etiology".

The Doctrine of Specific Etiology

As mentioned, the goal of both medicine and public health is, at least in part, to prevent or alleviate suffering caused by disease. Both disciplines adopt interventionist approaches to identify factors with "causal control" over disease outcomes. These factors, when removed, prevent disease onset. Ross, influenced by James Woodward, defines causal control as follows:

(I) X has causal control over Y if and only if an intervention that changes the value of X (and no other variable) in background circumstances B results in a change in the value of Y (Ross 2018, p. 6).

The first criterion for considering a cause of disease is thus causal control. Monocausal models such as Robert Koch's, in addition to (I), assume only one factor satisfies this condition:

(S1): For a given instance of disease D a single factor C causes D in the sense of (I) (Ross 2018, p. 8).

Whilst oxygen is necessary for TB, it is not a cause because it lacks causal control over the disease outcome, influencing only the patient's survival. The problem for the monocausal model arises when diseases have multiple causes meeting the causal control condition. This can be seen in the case of Phenylketonuria, which involves both genetic and dietary components. To address this, Ross introduces "shared etiology".

(S2): for all instances of disease D the same factor C or the same combination of factors (C1, C2,…Cn) cause every instance of D in the sense of (I) (Ross 2018, p. 12).

However, diseases such as Parkinson's fail to meet S2. The condition lacks a consistent set of causal factors. Similarly, causal factors are often unspecified (or at least, not well-specified) with psychiatric disorders, leading Ross to distinguish between "valid" or "legitimate" disease categories and "provisional" ones. Psychiatric conditions, identified primarily by symptoms, remain provisional until shared etiology is discovered. For Parkinson's, Ross suggests a distinction between "valid" diseases and diseases with a "provisional status" until a unifying shared etiology is found.

The doctrine of specific etiology preserves the benefits of the post-germ theory understanding of disease etiology without insisting on a single causal factor for all diseases. In this way, it is preferable to both the sufficient-cause model and the standard monocausal approach.

Now let us revisit the three questions posed regarding the sufficient cause model: whether it accurately reflects the nature of disease causation; how public health policy can be shaped by such models; and whether the approach reflects how medicine and public health identify causes.

Whereas the sufficient cause model has at least some ontological commitments: most notably, determinism about disease etiology, the doctrine of specific etiology does not. It's perfectly compatible with both deterministic and chancy disease causation. Whilst the analysis is prescriptive in some respects (particularly demarcating valid and provisional disease status), it is concerned with the concept of causation in the context of disease, not the ontology thereof. Of course, from an ontological perspective, the presence of oxygen *does* contribute in some way to the onset of all pathologies. But since this is an exercise in (prescriptive) conceptual analysis, this consequence is not concerning for the proponent of the doctrine of specific etiology.

The sufficient cause model requires the public health researcher to do some additional work when identifying which causes to focus on for preventative and curative interventions. One must identify which of the *inus* conditions are present in every sufficient cause, and which are manipulable. With the doctrine of specific etiology, this work is built into identifying the causes in the first place. According to the doctrine of specific etiology, an exposure only counts as a cause of disease if it has causal control over the outcome. The medical researcher thus knows immediately, once they have the causes identified by the doctrine of specific etiology, which causes are worthy of intervention: all of them.

Finally, the doctrine of specific etiology seems far closer to the actual use of "cause" within medicine and public health than the sufficient cause model. According to the latter, the presence of oxygen is a cause of all diseases. Under the doctrine of specific etiology, the presence of oxygen is not a cause of e.g. TB, but exposure to *Myobacterium tuberculosis* is. From the perspective of (even prescriptive) conceptual analysis, this is a considerable advantage.

In short, the doctrine of specific etiology has numerous advantages over the sufficient cause model. The causes it identifies *ex hypothesi* have causal control over disease-outcomes, guiding medical research and practice; it is more reflective of the actual practice of medicine and public health, and its accuracy does not depend on the assumption of determinism. Whilst the doctrine of specific etiology is not monocausal, it retains the core benefits of the monocausal approach, without falling foul of the obvious objections.

In the next section I consider the ontological aspects of disease etiology, both in the medical and public health context, in more detail.

4.3 The Ontology of Disease Etiology: Humeanism Vs Dispositionalism

Some philosophers of medicine and metaphysicians have argued that one's ontological assumptions can make a substantive difference to the treatment of patients. Mumford and Anjum (2011) contend that contemporary practices in epidemiology and medicine have led to Humean assumptions in mainstream medicine. This, in turn, has led to a one-size-fits-all approach to clinical practice. They argue that our unique physiologies, environments, habits, and preferences, mean that humans can react differently to the same treatment plan. This is trivially true, from the clinician's perspective. Just because a treatment worked on one patient does not imply it will work on another. But their worry runs deeper than that.

Clinical trials and other data collected over time provide doctors and their patients with determinations of risk. Risk, in epidemiology, is a purely statistical matter. It is a matter of association, not causation. To say that the ten-year lung cancer risk of a 68 year-old who's smoked two packets a day for 50 years is 15%, is just to say (or estimate using predictive models) that 15% of 68 year-olds who've smoked two packets a day for 50 years get lung cancer within 10 years (Bach et al. 1995). This reduces to 11% if they stop smoking immediately. Of course, there is a causal relationship between smoking and lung cancer, but one can meaningfully speak of the increased risk of lung cancer from drinking alcohol. More heavy drinkers die of lung cancer than non-drinkers. Alcohol does not cause lung cancer, but when smokers drink alcohol they tend to smoke more, so there's an increased absolute risk of lung cancer among those smokers who binge drink (Toriola et al. 2009).

The problem, so far as those sympathetic to Mumford and Anjum see it, is that medical practice acts on the assumption that e.g. every 68 year-old who continues to smoke two packets a day is 4% more likely to get lung cancer than those who stop. But this is not the case. Some will inevitably get lung cancer whether they stop or not.

I discussed evidence based medicine (EBM) and evidence based public health (EBPH) at length in Chap. 3. There, I noted Rocca and Anjum (2020) objection to "treating patients as statistics" when they all have unique dispositions, but did not elaborate on the ontological underpinnings of their claims. That is work for this chapter.

Rocca and Anjum argue that EBM is grounded by a Humean approach to causation. This thought is echoed by Roger Kerry et al. in their paper "Causation and Evidence Based Practice: an ontological review" (Kerry et al. 2012). Whilst extensive exploration of Humean causation is beyond the scope of this book, Humeans are paradigmatic empiricists; David Hume believed one should "proportion one's belief to the evidence". Humeans further contend that "necessary connection" in the objects is fundamentally unobservable (indeed, Hume's brand of empiricism leads him to take "necessary connection in the objects" to be meaningless). Agents see one event, followed by another. That is all. There is no observable "necessary connection in the objects" in addition, even when the sequence is genuinely causal.

Observers do, however, recognize patterns of events of one type being followed by events of another—events of type B regularly occurring subsequent to events of type A. When this kind of regularity is observed (constant conjunction), alongside temporal priority of A to B, and contiguity (the objects involved in these events touch), we form a habit of mind connecting events of type A to events to events of type B. Our intuition that events of type B are necessitated by events of type A (the feeling that token event B *has* to occur after observing token event A) arises from these features, and for Hume, that belief is the final ingredient required for a causal inference.

Strictly speaking, very few causal relationships in medicine or public health fulfil the criteria of this formula. Constant conjunction is a rarity. Not all smokers get cancer, but smoking causes cancer. However, the essence of Humeanism remains in the causal inferences drawn by the health sciences. Causal inferences are made by observing regularities, albeit not exceptionless ones.

Counterfactuals

In addition to the regularity definition provided above, Hume adds: "Or in other words where, if the first object had never been, the second never had existed" (Hume 1748 (2007), VIII, p. 56). This is a counterfactual conditional, but whilst the "Or in other words" remark suggests it's similar in content to the regularity approach, it quite clearly is not. More recent Humeans, most notably David Lewis (1973), have rejected Hume's regularity approach. They focus almost exclusively on the counterfactual analysis (or refined versions thereof). The health sciences have done the same thing.

The core of interventionism is understanding what would happen were one to interfere in a particular way. But whilst Lewis's account of causation concerns singular causation (crudely: event A caused event B if and only if A and B occurred, and if A had not occurred, B would not have occurred), the health sciences are typically more interested in general causal claims (do events of type A cause events of type B?). In both the singular and general cases, the following question arises: how does one assess the counterfactual scenario? After all, *ex hypothesi* the counterfactual scenario never occurs.

For Lewis, one compares what occurs in the actual world with what occurs in the closest possible world in which the prospective cause does not obtain—a world which matches the actual world in terms of the state of affairs prior to the prospective cause's occurrence in the actual world (Lewis 1973). One then applies the laws of nature of the actual world to the possible world, to infer what would happen had the prospective cause not obtained. But when Bob gets cancer, we can't see what would have happened had he never smoked. So how do epidemiologists assess the counterfactuals they're interested in?

There are at least two ways in which public health researchers address important counterfactual questions (such as: "would fewer people get lung cancer if fewer people smoked?", or "would fewer people die of COVID-19 were everyone vaccinated?"). The first is through the clinical trials. These come in a number of forms, including randomized controlled trials, cohort studies, case-control studies, and so on. I discussed these in Chap. 3, and won't repeat myself, here. However, what they all have in common is the comparison between a control group and an exposure group. Ideally, the exact same cohort of participants would be in both the exposure and control groups at the same time. That way we could guarantee the truth of the counterfactual in question. That's impossible (nobody can be in both the exposure and control groups), but by comparing groups of similar people (through randomization) with different exposures, researchers are (at least in principle) able to make quantified estimates of the effect of a given exposure, as well as to specify a P-value; that is, to specify the probability of the null-hypothesis—that the observed difference between the exposure and control group is the result of chance, not the exposure.

The second strategy concerning counterfactuals is known as "The Potential Outcomes Approach" (POA). POA process is similar to that Lewis adopts in some respects, but very different in others. The POA is concerned with many "potential outcomes" (whereby outcomes can be a number of variables, including incidence rates, life expectancy, and so on), the values of which are determined through (a) actual group studies, and (b) estimates of the outcomes of counterfactual studies; not only whether or not the actual outcome occurs given the non-occurrence of the actual exposure, but specific data concerning outcomes under a number of possible contrary-to-fact exposures. The strategy thus runs roughly as follows:

There are a number of possible actions, only one of which is actual. Take the actual action of an individual or population to be *x0*, and all alternative exposures to that individual or population to be uniquely specified: *x1, x2, x3,* and so on.

1. Take O to be a measure of outcome, and O*(x0)* to be the outcome of the observable event *x0.* O*(xn)* for all values of *n* except *0* are unobservable—they are the counterfactual outcomes. All outcomes O*(xn)* are potential outcomes.
2. Compare the actual outcome O(*x0*) with any one counterfactual outcome O(*xc*), to measure the effect of *x0* versus O(*xc*)

Outcomes other than O*(x0)* are contrary-to-fact and thus unobservable, but reasonable estimation (assuming this is possible) of these values admits of numerous effect-measures (for example, if one takes *x0* to be "immunised against yellow fever", and *x1* to be "not immunised against yellow fever", one can calculate the risk of yellow fever ratio due to non-immunisation versus immunisation by O*(x1)*/O*(x0)*).

Note here a further important difference between the Lewisian conception of causation and the POA; namely, that the strategy employed implies that it is meaningless to assert that "non-immunisation is a cause *simpliciter* of yellow fever"—one must first determine which intervention/action it's relative to (Dammann and Smart 2019). One must assert that "non-immunisation causes yellow fever *versus immunization*". Unprotected penile-vaginal sex (where HIV is prevalent) therefore *is* a cause of HIV versus abstinence, but is *not* a cause of HIV versus unprotected anal sex (where HIV is prevalent). Relative to unprotected anal sex, unprotected penile-vaginal sex reduces risk of HIV.

Clinical trials and the POA can result in general causal claims: smoking causes cancer (versus not smoking); a vaccine reduces risk of mortality (versus no vaccine); statins reduce risk of myocardial infarction (versus no statin), and so on. As noted above, whilst the core tenets of Hume's account of causation will rarely be fully met in the public health context, the counterfactual approaches adopted by medicine and public health remain broadly Humean insofar as the counterfactual inferences are grounded by regularities. Kerry *et al* write:

> Health science seems not to claim that causation is itself observable. It is only the regularities of one event being followed by another that is observable. In Humean terms, health science has no concern with understanding causes as anything more than regularities. That is, there is nothing internal to the causal process, which relates to a cause producing an effect, for example some sort of real force or compulsion. Causation is just one thing followed regularly by another. Although neo-Humeans are happy with this stance as a complete account of causation, health science and practice might not be. Health science in one sense seems rich with a history of informative science ranging from laboratory studies through to large-scale clinical trials. Further, health care itself is constructed of clinical experiences, patient values and presentations. If a Humean stance is to be taken, which seems the only plausible philosophical account of causation in health science so far, then what is there to be said of remaining knowledge, experiences and patient input? The [Evidence Based Practice (EBP)] framework determines that clinical decisions – entailing causal intentions – should integrate as much of this knowledge as possible. A Humean commitment seems not to allow such background conditions a role in the understanding of a precise nature of causation in health care. (Kerry et al. 2012, p. 1008)

This is arguably a straw man characterization of EBM and the corresponding EBP framework, however. Clinical experience is reflected both in the EBM and later EBPH hierarchies (albeit lower down than clinical trials), and the importance of considering patients as unique individuals is highlighted in Sacket et al's own commentary on EBM:

> The practice of evidence based medicine means integrating individual clinical expertise with the best available external clinical evidence from systematic research. By individual clinical expertise we mean the proficiency and judgment that individual clinicians acquire through clinical experience and clinical practice… Without clinical expertise, practice risks becoming tyrannised by evidence, for even excellent external evidence may be inapplicable to or inappropriate for an individual patient. (Sackett et al. 1996, pp. 71–72)

Evidence based practitioners want clinical decisions based on appropriate evidence, but not at the cost of ignoring patient-values, individual patient needs, and so on. The fact that the upper echelons of the EBM hierarchy take a broadly Humean approach to identifying causal relationships doesn't prevent that. That being said, whilst Kerry et al's critique of EBP might be unduly harsh, the alternative ontological framework they propose as a replacement for this Humean approach is worthy of consideration—both from the perspective of clinical medicine, and public health. They suggest a dispositional ontology:

> In causal dispositionalism, a cause does not necessitate its effect, but rather tends towards it. Smoking disposes or tends towards cancer, but not everyone who smokes gets cancer. A tendency can be stronger or weaker. Low-rate occurrences of causal connections are better understood from this dispositional account. The account has little interest in causal partners being considered as discrete events, that is a 'cause' and an 'effect'. Rather, partners interact with each other with far greater intimacy and simultaneity than the Humean account allows. An effect is manifested when there is sufficient interaction of mutually accountable causal partners. Immediately, the patient becomes of utmost importance in the causal process. (Kerry et al. 2012, p. 1010)

Kerry et al. claim that "low-rate occurrences of causal connections are better understood[2] from this dispositional account". It's worth distinguishing between understanding causal connections and identifying them. In terms of identifying causal relationships, the current strategies

[2] My emphasis.

seem to do a reasonable job at the population level, even when the effect-size is small. A recent systematic review and meta-analysis investigating the effectiveness of statins revealed, for example, that statins reduced absolute risk of all-cause mortality by 0.8%, and of myocardial infarction by 1.3% (Byrne et al. 2022). The effect size is small, but significant (in the sense that the P value is less than 0.05). It indicates that rolling statins out to large quantities of people could save many lives, despite reducing absolute risk only marginally. Kerry et al. might argue, however, that identifying causal relationships and understanding them are not the same thing. Perhaps a better understanding of statins would enable medical practitioners to better identify those who statins will genuinely help, saving millions from a lifetime of taking medication that will not help them.

Dispositions in Disease Etiology, Prevention, and Treatment

Following Werkhoven (Werkhoven 2019, p. 934) and Nordenfelt (2018), I argued in Chap. 1. that health could be understood at the level of physiological parts, organisms, and populations in terms of their capacities. From an ontological perspective, Mumford and Anjum take a similar approach to disease etiology. They propose a vectors approach to model causal dispositionalism, where each vector represents a real dispositional property. In the medical context, these properties tend the patient towards certain health outcomes when the corresponding stimulus conditions are met. They are properties of both the patient and (where relevant) the exposure.

Each vector has a directedness towards a particular outcome and a specified magnitude. That outcome might be the initial contraction of the disease (illness causation), or a well-specified symptom (post-pathomechanisms). The final dispositional outcome is reflected by the resultant vector—the sum value of all those factors that dispose one towards and away from the specified outcome.

The magnitude of the resultant vectors (a function of the dispositions of both the patient and the exposure) and the type of disposition represented by the vectors, vary from one individual to another, avoiding the "one-size-fits-all" assumptions of the Humean ontology. In other words, whilst epidemiological studies can demonstrate that at the population-level, diets high in saturated fats or genetic preconditions can increase risk of myocardial infarction, the magnitude of the dispositional vector towards (or away from) myocardial infarction provided by these factors (the real metaphysical probabilities) cannot be calculated through a frequentist approach. The vector models are unique to each patient.

Given the nature of vectors, one might plausibly introduce a multi-dimensional model, reflecting a plurality of health outcomes. For example, penicillin is disposed both to kill bacteria, and to cause auto-immune reactions. The size of the vector towards causing an auto-immune reaction will depend on the dispositions (allergies) of the patient. Whilst it remains difficult to measure dispositions (despite advances in genetic research), I deem the model appealing. It treats every patient as a unique individual in a way that EBM cannot.

The pathomechanisms leading from illness causation to the onset of clinical disease are unquestionably complex, involving significant interaction with the patient's unique physiology. Rather than simply describing what percentage of patients will manifest disease given the exposure, or what percentage will recover given an intervention, the dispositional vector model provides an ontological *explanation* for why certain patients react well to treatments and others do not. The vectors represent metaphysically real dispositional properties. Understanding these processes and acting appropriately; that is, basing one's interventions on the unique dispositions of patients, rather than prescribing the same intervention to all patients with the same pathological condition (although, again, it's worth noting that EBP does not suggest this), should have favourable health outcomes.

4.4 The Dispositional Vector Model and Public Health

The examples in Sect. 4.3. pertain to clinical medicine. The vectors discussed represent the dispositional characteristics of individual patients. However, the model can be adapted to apply to populations. Just as an individual patient might be disposed to react violently to certain stimuli (due to e.g. some mental illness or substance abuse), or manifest specific symptoms given exposure to a particular pathogen, so a population can have the emergent disposition to react violently to certain stimuli (e.g. a propensity to protest violently in reaction to some political situation or food insecurity).

Due to differences in socioeconomic conditions, environmental factors such as climate, and aggregated genetic differences at the population level, different populations have different emergent dispositions. Age distributions between populations can vary widely. The same applies to levels of obesity, poverty, nutrition, and so on. These differences correspond to different vulnerabilities, and importantly from the perspective of public health, different needs. It is the job of those working in public health to identify these needs and provide cost-effective interventions to meet them. Just as the vector model can provide tailored guidance for appropriate interventions for individuals, so awareness of the population's dispositions can guide public health policymakers regarding appropriate public health interventions (and how to prepare for interventions that might be needed in future).

The dispositions and capacities of populations are (weakly) emergent properties. They emerge from the dispositions of those that comprise the population, their interpersonal relationships, and the environment. These, in turn, depend on a wide variety of circumstances ranging from socioeconomic circumstances to religious and/or political belief systems. Although these population-level macro-dispositions are reducible to those of their parts, they are difficult to predict. Consider, for example, a population's susceptibility to a particular epidemic; one caused by an airborne pathogen such as TB, for which an effective vaccine is available. This susceptibility can be cashed out in terms of dispositions and my preferred means of measuring the health of a population: to what extent would the capacities of the population be negatively affected were the infection introduced to the population? In other words, how is the population disposed to react when there is a TB outbreak—will an epidemic ensue or not?

The answer will differ from one population to another. TB affects patients with comorbidities such as HIV more than others (Sonnenberg et al. 2004). The percentage of the population vaccinated against the disease makes a difference. The population's access to hospitals and clinics makes a difference. A healthy, vaccinated population with easy access to high quality healthcare is far less susceptible to TB than a largely unvaccinated population with a high HIV prevalence in a region with poor healthcare. This population-scale scenario can be modelled using vectors in a similar way to that discussed in Sect. 4.3. Only, instead of the individual, the model represents a population, and instead of disease-status, the model represents epidemic-status.

Figure 4.2 is a crude, inaccurate, and incomplete representation of TB, but it illustrates the concept. Public health policymakers can dispose populations away from epidemics (speaking more broadly than just TB) by introducing clean water supplies, providing access to high quality medical care, ensuring the population has easy access to vaccines and nutritious foods, ensuring wastewater is properly treated, and so on.

As is the case with individual patients, some causal factors are more easily interfered with than others. A high median age disposes a

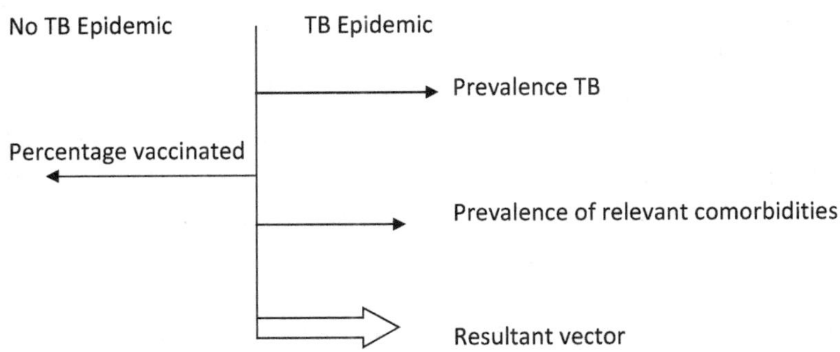

Fig. 4.2 Simplified vector model of dispositions in public health (TB epidemic)

population towards worse health outcomes with e.g. COVID-19, but that's not something government can easily interfere with. They can, however, impose lockdowns that reduce close contacts, introduce efficient vaccination programmes, and so on. All this can be reflected on the vector model.

The vector model can be expanded from transmissible disease epidemics to other areas of concern within public health. Now let us consider two further kinds of public health issue. The first also concerns health problems caused by pathogens, but in this case, the disease is spread as a result of inadequate infrastructure. The second involves no pathogens; a chronic disease caused primarily by lifestyle (predominantly diet and exercise) and genetic preconditions. Whilst the three kinds of public health issue discussed here are not exhaustive, I hope to demonstrate that they share a common metaphysical causal framework, and are ontologically similar in relevant respects. Ultimately, I suggest that Mumford and Anjum's dispositional etiological framework may be generalizable to (at least, many) public health issues.

Water Infrastructure

However one measures the health of populations, it's clear that population health has broadly improved over time—radically over the last two hundred years or so. Child mortality rates have plummeted globally, and life expectancy has increased by a matter of decades (Liou et al. 2020). It might be tempting to put this down largely to improvements in medicine: germ theory, the discovery of antibiotics, advancements in surgery and cancer treatments, and so forth. Whilst advances in medicine certainly contribute to the improvement in life expectancy and population health more generally, arguably a greater contribution has been made by improvements to water and sanitation infrastructure, as well as dietary improvements. Bartram et al., for example, note that:

> 88% of diarrhoeal disease—the second leading cause of death in children younger than five years after respiratory illnesses—is attributed to unsafe drinking water, inadequate sanitation, and poor hygiene. Diarrhoea mor-

> bidity is reduced by around 21% through improved water supply and by around 37% through improved sanitation. (Bartram et al. 2005)

An ontological account of public health interventions would be incomplete if it focused purely on medical interventions. Public health interventions go beyond vaccine programmes and the treatment of disease. They include all measures designed to improve human health, and that includes the provision of clean water and adequate sanitation.

I propose here that the same dispositional causal ontological framework used for infectious disease epidemics can be adopted for public health interventions focused on infrastructure. Consider cholera, a waterborne bacterial infection.

Cholera epidemics typically occur in places with high levels of poverty and inadequate access to clean water. The bacteria pass out of infected individuals through fecal matter, which then contaminates a common water supply, leading to further infections. If patients with cholera receive prompt medical attention, the mortality rate is less than 1%. However, left untreated, the mortality rate rapidly rises to 50%-70% (Kuna and Gajewski 2017); perhaps unsurprisingly, a lack of access to clean water is often associated with a lack of easy access to quality healthcare.

The dispositional approach can be applied to cholera just as easily as TB. The public health interventions, despite not being strictly medical in nature, play a similar role when it comes to fixing the magnitude of the vectors involved. In this instance, the presence of well-maintained water infrastructure is the difference between a contaminated and non-contaminated water supply(Figs. 4.3 and 4.4).

Eliminating the contaminated water removes the primary cause of the cholera epidemic, "tending" the population away from manifesting a cholera epidemic.

Obesity and Type 2 Diabetes

The previous examples of TB and cholera both concern infectious diseases. But many diseases have genetic causes and/or environmental causes with no associated pathogen.

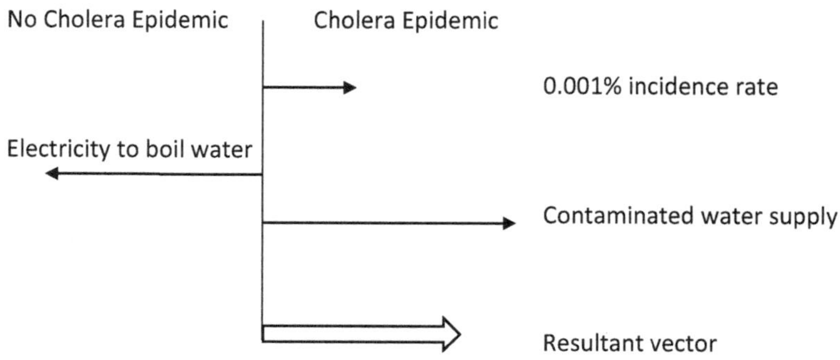

Fig. 4.3 Vector model of dispositions for cholera epidemic—no clean water

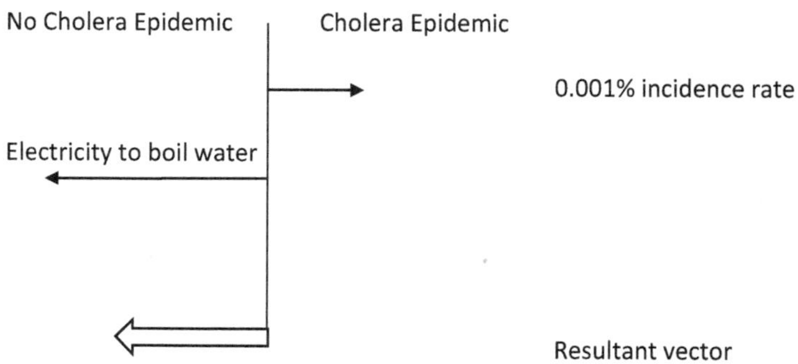

Fig. 4.4 Vector model of dispositions for cholera epidemic—clean water

Obesity has been recognized by the World Health Organization as an epidemic since 1997. Whilst the both the disease-status of obesity, and whether it can meaningfully be considered a cause of disease/mortality (Hernan and Taubman 2008) remains a matter of debate, the capacities approach endorsed in this book would likely support its disease-status (certainly if disease is to be understood as substantive reductions in health). In some instances, obesity restricts a patient's capacities in a plethora of ways, from placing limitations on cardiovascular exercise, to, in extreme cases, an inability to bathe oneself. Obesity is also risk-factor for myocardial infarction, type 2 diabetes, and many other pathological conditions. Despite not being recognized as a cause of type 2 diabetes, obese patients have a significantly higher risk of developing the condition.

The obesity epidemic first appeared in the United States between 1976 and 1980, then spread across the Global North. Prevalence grew in the US from 15% in 1976–1980, to 30.9% in 1999–2000 (Temple 2022), and has continued to grow. For the 2017–2020 period, obesity in the US stood at 41.9% (CDC 2022). It is not restricted to the developed world, however. It is estimated that 115 million people in developing countries are clinically obese (Ellulu et al. 2014).

Social determinants of health play the dominant role in the obesity epidemic. The economically disadvantaged are at significantly higher risk, since nutritious healthy food options are typically more expensive than foods high in carbohydrates and saturated fats (Drewnowski 2012). Access to healthy foods is also often more difficult for disadvantaged communities. Whereas nearly every poor urban area will have a cheap fast-food outlet, green grocers are more frequently located in affluent areas. Healthy foods are thus less accessible to the poor. Unhealthy foods are also marketed far more aggressively than their healthier counterparts. Targeted advertisements for fast food brands are commonplace, but it's rare to see fruits and vegetables advertised in a similar way.

Although no pathogen is involved in the spread of obesity, the same metaphysical approach to both the disease etiology of obesity, and the ontology of an obesity epidemic (to be discussed in Sect. 4.5), can be adopted as for transmissible diseases. Its social determinants can be mapped onto a dispositional vector diagram (Figs. 4.5 and 4.6).

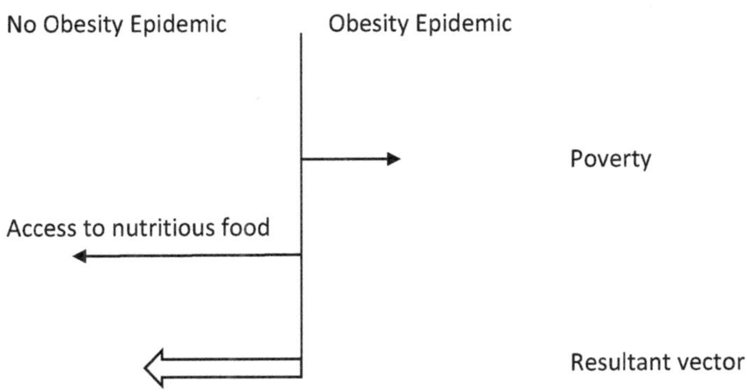

Fig. 4.5 Vector model of dispositions for obesity epidemic—low poverty

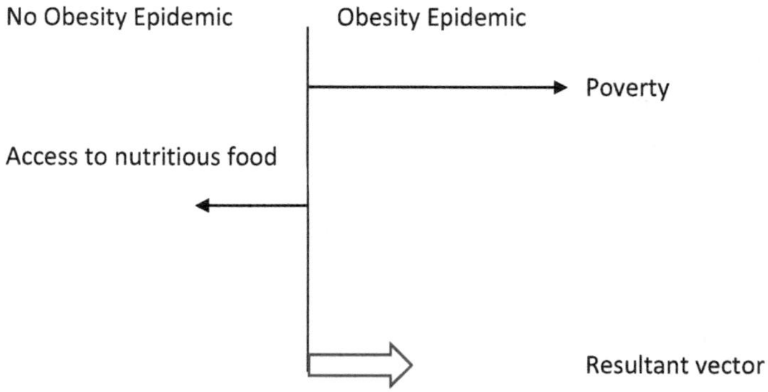

Fig. 4.6 Vector model of dispositions for obesity epidemic—low poverty

Poverty disposes individuals within populations towards obesity, as does a lack of access to healthy nutritious foods. To some extent, these social determinants are manipulable. Poverty is difficult, albeit not impossible to address over time through economic growth, but nutrition education programmes can have a measurable effect on obesity levels, as can legislative and economic interventions such as sugar taxes.

Populations, like individuals, are unique. Their unique contexts and the unique make-up of their populations dispose them towards different health outcomes given the same exposures. As discussed in the previous chapter, evidence based public health is cognizant of this, and warns public health policymakers to tailor their interventions to the population in question. I argued in the previous chapter that, all too often (as with the COVID-19 pandemic), one-size-fits-all interventions are globally recommended by recognized institutions. Consideration of the dispositional model above could help policymakers identify the best interventions for their unique populations, carefully selecting those that maximize population-level capacities that optimally promote opportunities for individuals to improve their health.

Naturally, policymaking requires evaluation of more than one dispositional vector model. In addition to considering the risk of an epidemic, policymakers must identify and evaluate the effect of their interventions on as many health outcomes as possible. In this way, policymakers can reduce the risk and/or impact of epidemics, without exposing the population to other forms of harm. Of course, the emergent dispositions of populations may not be what we predict them to be. Our models will reflect our epistemic position, and that may not match up with the ontological reality. One of the tasks of public health is to produce models that match this reality as closely as possible.

In this section I have discussed the metaphysics of disease etiology, ending with the dispositional vector model applied to epidemic-status. I take epidemics to be an emergent property of populations. In the next section, I outline this ontological conception in more detail.

4.5 The Ontology of Epidemics

Given the implications for public health policy, particularly regarding the availability of emergency funding, it is important for governments to be able to promptly identify both the beginnings of new epidemics, as well as their endings. Miss the beginning by too wide a margin, and many interventions (such as lockdown) become less effective, or entirely ineffective. Miss the end, and governments can waste billions. Healthcare economics is a critical part of public health. Every cent spent on one issue, is money that can't be spent on another.

According to the Centers for Disease Control (CDC), "Epidemic refers to an increase, often sudden, in the number of cases of a disease above what is normally expected in that population in that area" (CDC 2022). This is a purely biostatistical matter. The end of epidemics is more nuanced. Erika Charters and Kristin Heitman contend that "Epidemics end once the disease becomes accepted into people's daily lives and routines, becoming endemic-domesticated-and accepted" (Charters and Heitman 2021, p. 218). This is subjectivist in character. So there is an asymmetry between the beginnings and ends of epidemics. The beginnings are determined through a value-free and objectivist strategy, the ends are inherently value-laden and subjectivist.

I have argued (with Herculaas Combrink) elsewhere for a prescriptive account of epidemics that helps reconcile this disconnect. We propose a value-dependent realist ontology of epidemics, according to which the degree to which the disease has been accepted within a population plays little-to-no role in the ending of an epidemic (Smart and Combrink 2022). Similarly, whilst the current CDC definition of epidemic makes no reference to harm, we argue in favour of a value-laden approach to both the beginnings and endings of epidemics.

The existing classificatory system, we argue, is flawed. In large part because a disease can become "accepted into people's daily lives and routines" long before the epidemic should be declared over. The HIV epidemic in South Africa is a good example of this. South Africa is home to around one in five of those infected with HIV, globally (Burger et al. 2022), with roughly 10% of the population receiving Antiretroviral Therapy (ART). The epidemic begun in the late 1980s, and HIV testing and treatment is something South Africans are very used to. But despite its prevalence, and despite its being accepted as a part of South Africans' daily routine, the disease still causes tremendous harm. Alongside the related TB casualties, it's one of the country's leading causes of mortality. Even if it weren't still causing deaths (perhaps due to a perfect ART programme), it would still be causing harm. HIV positive patients often spend an entire day waiting in a queue for their ART medication. They must obtain this once a month, and access to the clinics is not always easy for those living in remote areas.

Epidemic status attracts major funding. Were the epidemic declared over (it hasn't been, and is unlikely to be any time soon), and the funding cut, this would be disasterous for the millions of South Africans living with HIV. Since the HIV epidemic has not, in fact, been declared over, on the face of it Charters and Heitman's account is descriptively false. The end of an epidemic is declared when the disease is no longer considered a significant threat to public health, rather than when the population have made it a part of their daily routines.

The ontology of epidemics should reflect the role harm plays in epidemics. Epidemic status in a population, we argue, is an emergent property of a complex system—the population. But when does a population instantiate this property? Whilst observing the early stages of an outbreak can help predict the likelihood of a future epidemic, we think the harm caused by the disease in question should be central to this property. Providing a symmetrical model, whereby both the beginning and end of an epidemic is contingent on a harm-threshold being breached, provides both a qualitative parsimony to the model, and an intuitive understanding of the effect a disease is having on the population in question.

We propose a value-dependent realist account. Most value-dependent accounts in the philosophy of medicine are subjectivist in character. The value criterion in Wakefield's (1992) account of mental dysfunction, for example, specifies that diseases must be disvalued *by the patient's society*. Cooper's (2002) account of disease specifies that for a condition to be a disease, it must be considered a "bad thing to have" *by the patient herself*. However, the notion of harm need not be subjectivist. In moral philosophy, for example, moral realists depend on an objective notion of harm. Something can be "bad" irrespective of the subjective opinions of members of the population. It is this realist sense of harm that we employ. For a disease in a population to reach epidemic status, it must cause a certain degree of harm to the population as a complex system: an objective, mind-independent degree of harm must be caused, which crosses a certain threshold. The threshold itself may be difficult to identify, in the same way that it's difficult to identify when a man becomes bald. But we appeal to an epistemic account of vagueness. We may not know precisely when the threshold is breached, but it's nonetheless a mind-independent matter of fact. That said, just as we can more-or-less identify bald people without too much difficulty, we can identify epidemics. Following my capacities approach to measuring the health of populations, the degree of harm should be estimated by evaluating the loss of capacities across the populations.

Contrast two, year-long scenarios for some infectious disease D. Suppose that during this year, there are two waves of infections. In the first scenario there is no intervention. Once the harm caused by D rises above the proposed "epidemic threshold", turning from an outbreak into an epidemic, it doesn't retrace below that threshold for at least a year. It dips between the peaks of the two waves of infections, but never drops below the threshold. In scenario one, the harm corresponds with the number of cases (though this needn't be the case).

In the second scenario, we assume the same caseload, but this time with an intervention at the peak of the first wave. The intervention is ineffective at preventing the spread of D, but effective at reducing the harm D causes. It is not uncommon for vaccines to have such an effect.

Indeed, arguably this happened during the COVID-19 pandemic. In the second scenario, the intervention reduces the harm caused by D below the harm threshold, and it stays below that threshold, even when the caseload starts to increase as wave two begins. In this second scenario, the disease has become endemic. If in the future, the level of harm caused by D were to rise above the threshold, which it could, were the vaccine to lose its effectiveness, D would regain epidemic status. Thus despite becoming endemic, D remains an "epidemicable" disease (it has the potential to become an epidemic).

In this section I presented an ontological account of epidemics as an emergent property of a complex system—one grounded by the objective degree of harm (observable through loss of capacities) it causes that population. Although an outbreak only becomes an epidemic once that harm threshold is breached, public health policymakers must attempt to prevent that from occurring. Identifying disease outbreaks before they become epidemics is central to this project, as is taking preventative measures, such as vaccine programmes. Similarly, it's important that the end of an epidemic is correctly and timeously identified. Failure to do so can have serious health consequences, as government's limited resources might continue to be allocated to an issue that should no longer be a priority.

4.6 Conclusions

In this chapter I have addressed various issues within the metaphysics of public health, from conceptual analysis in disease etiology to the ontology of epidemics. Following Edout I propose a three-stage model of disease etiology for transmissible diseases, adding pathogen origination to illness causation and pathomechanisms. From the conceptual analysis perspective of disease causation, I considered and rejected the monocausal model. Rather than accepting traditional multifactorial analyses such as Rothman's sufficient cause model, I endorse Ross's doctrine of specific etiology. This admits of the core motivations behind Koch's postulates, whilst allowing for diseases to have more than one cause.

In the second half of the chapter, I considered the ontology of disease etiology, comparing Humean approaches with dispositional accounts. The dispositionalists reject the Humean approaches central to EBM on the grounds that individual patients have unique sets of dispositions. One should not, they argue, project population-level responses to interventions onto individual patients. This kind of objection is less potent against public health policy making, since population-level responses are precisely what policymakers are interested in. However, I demonstrate that the dispositional models are just as applicable to public health crisis as they are to individual instances of disease.

I conclude with a value-dependent realist ontological account of epidemics. This, I suggest, is an improvement on the subjectivist account proposed by Charters and Heitman, first because of its parsimonious symmetry, and second because it more accurately reflects when substantive interventions should cease.

5

An Introduction to Public Health Ethics

5.1 Outline

Public health policymaking, like medical practice, has a substantive impact on people's lives: their wellbeing, life-expectancy, and even liberty. There is thus an extensive ethical dimension to public health policymaking. Policies that enhance the health of one person or group might do so at the expense of others. The reality of health economics ensures this is almost always the case. Furthermore, policies can either respect the autonomy of those affected, or entirely ignore it. They might increase or reduce health inequalities.

Public health ethics is intertwined with the goals of public health discussed in Chap. 2. I noted there that the traditional goal of public health is simply to improve the health of populations (however that is to be interpreted), but further that egalitarian considerations have come to the fore in recent years. I suggested that should one adopt the capacities approach to measuring health, and direct public health policy to improving population-level capacities, the egalitarian desiderata would naturally be accommodated. In this chapter and the next I develop that idea. I consider a number of approaches to public health ethics, ultimately (in

B. Smart, *The Philosophy of Public Health*,
https://doi.org/10.1007/978-3-031-98804-2_5

Chap. 6) leading to a defense of what I call "capacities-based principlism".

In Sect. 5.2. I present and critique the utilitarian/welfarist approach to public health ethics. Applying John Stuart Mill's initial formulation entails focusing on the promotion of utility, traditionally measured through net happiness: crudely, maximizing pleasure and minimizing pain (although alternative measures of welfare can be adopted in the public health context). I highlight some general problems with this approach, including egalitarian concerns, and further suggest that whilst appeal to happiness is at least a part of identifying the vital goals (see Chap. 2), using it as one's sole measure can lead to additional health inequalities.

Having rejected the utilitarian/welfarist approach, in Sect. 5.3 I consider (and suggest the adoption of) some of John Rawls's conclusions in *A Theory of Justice* (Rawls 1999). Although extensive discussion of the thought experiment informing his fundamental principles of justice is beyond the scope of this chapter, I outline the basic argument, and ultimately endorse the principles of liberty, equality and fraternity (due to the gendered nature of "fraternity", I prefer "solidarity" and will use that term outside of quotation) that fall out of it. I then go on to view specific public health orientated ethical theories in terms of both their internal coherence, and their coherence with Rawlsian values.

In Sect. 5.4. I consider two principlist approaches to public health ethics (Childress et al. 2002; Kass 2001). Whilst I endorse a broadly principlist idea, the versions set out by Nancy Kass and Childress et al. lack sufficient detail. Kass sets out a useful process for making public health policy decisions, and Childress et al. some general moral considerations; but neither specify precisely which harms should be avoided and which benefits pursued. I nonetheless borrow a number of Childress et al.'s principles in capacities-based principlism, and largely endorse the six-step process Kass promotes. Finally, in Sect. 5.5. I present and critique Venkatapuram's capabilities approach to public health ethics (Venkantapuram 2013). Venkatapuram suggests that health itself is a meta-capability—the capability to realize Nussbaum's ten capabilities necessary for living a life worthy of human dignity (Nussbaum 2006). Naturally, this conception of human health lends itself to an account of public health ethics, since promoting health promotes dignity. I find much of Venkatapuram's work compelling, but argue (in this chapter and the next) that his approach can be improved and developed in a number of ways.

Each of the accounts considered in this chapter look at public health ethics purely in terms of the effect public health policy has on the individuals comprising the population; that is, they do not consider the effect on populations as complex systems. This sets the stage for the novel capacities approach to public health ethics presented and defended in Chap. 6, in which I suggest public health has duties both to the individuals comprising populations, and to populations as complex systems.

5.2 Utilitarianism and Public Health

The first approach to public health ethics considered in this chapter derives from Mill's consequentialism. Mill proposes that the right action is that which maximizes "utility", generally cashed out in terms of maximizing pleasure and minimizing pain.

> The creed which accepts as the foundation of morals, Utility, or the Greatest-Happiness Principle, holds that actions are right in proportion as they tend to promote happiness, wrong as they tend to produce the reverse of happiness. By happiness is intended pleasure, and the absence of pain; by unhappiness, pain, and the privation of pleasure. (Mill 1871, p. 9)

In health terms, this roughly translates to what Venkatapuram terms a "welfare theory of health", although whether welfare can truly be captured by pleasure and pain is a matter of debate.

This basic formulation of Mill's consequentialism is blind to whose welfare is improved or reduced by a policy decision or intervention. The policies should promote as much welfare as possible with the limited available resources. This provides some intuitively sensible results. Suppose one had ten million dollars. With that money, one could either upgrade water infrastructure (that desperately needs upgrading), helping prevent prevalent water-borne diseases severely affecting a million people, or one could buy ten MRI machines for public hospitals. Whilst the MRI machines are certainly useful, utility is maximized by using those funds in the way that benefit the most people to the greatest extent. The utilitarian approach, in this context, focuses on the efficient use of resources.

The basic principle of maximizing utility could be adjusted to accommodate a variety of metrics. Venkatapuram states that

> a welfarist approach to health would probably focus just on maximizing a single metric of health across individuals. And this health metric would be related to utility, some mental characteristic, such as pleasure, happiness, satisfaction or desire related to physical and mental functioning. In its simplest form, such a metric could be 'mortality cases averted'; there would be more utility from people living than if they were dead. (Venkantapuram 2013, p. 213)

I will not dwell on which measure would provide the best health outcomes for now (but note the discussion of QALYs and DALYs in Chap. 2. as possible alternatives), since the objection outlined below is equally troubling to all possible metrics.

Although efficiency is certainly important in public health, focusing only on maximizing pleasure and minimizing pain (or averting as many mortality cases as possible, or whatever metric one chooses) with the available resources is problematic from an egalitarian perspective. It might well, for example, be far more cost effective to focus one's health-investments in densely populated urban areas, ignoring the sparsely populated rural regions. It costs less to build one large hospital accessible to the millions living close by, than to build the scores of smaller clinics necessary to accommodate the same number of people scattered across sparsely populated rural villages. According to the welfarist/utilitarian strategy, we should always go for the most efficient option, but that would mean ignoring the health needs of those in rural areas.

Further, suppose one adopted "happiness", or "pleasure" as one's unit of utility. Then, exclusively providing treatment for and extending the lives of those who are currently ill, but otherwise living privileged happy lives, could provide a more favourable utility output than providing treatment and extending the lives of those who are struggling. This would only be true if happiness is correlated with wealth and privilege, but at least some studies suggest that it is—at least to an extent (Branchflower and Oswald 2011). The traditional utilitarian approach when applied to public health could thus serve to drive health inequalities.

Depending on which metric one employs, the utilitarian approach also has consequences for who would qualify for treatment in terms of age demographics. Should one use the "mortality cases averted" metric, it might maximize utility to focus public health interventions on extending the lives of the elderly, since they (on average) have the highest mortality risk. Change that metric to years of life lost, and the very elderly might never qualify for treatment. Better to treat younger people with long lives ahead of them. The same would apply to maximizing pleasure. Should one use Mill's preferred metrics of pleasure and pain, it also seems to follow that those likely to live the longest (from the moment of intervention) are more entitled to benefit from public health interventions e.g., during a deadly pandemic, than everyone else. Governments would have a greater responsibility to ensure a community of wealthy people with long life expectancies survive the pandemic, than a community of poor people who tend to die earlier. Finally, as noted in Chap. 2. in response to Brülde's measure of health, if one adopts "total utilitarianism" over its "average" alternative (whereby one considers total aggregated levels of happiness/welfare, rather than the average level per person), Parfit's (1984) repugnant conclusion could rear its ugly head in public health policy making.

Should one adopt the (total) utilitarian approach to public health ethics, it seems the primary concern could be to maximize the size of the population (ensuring only that their lives are at least minimally worth living). This could be achieved with "public health interventions" such as banning contraception, banning abortion, and so on. But surely it is better to have fewer people living a very high quality of life in good health, than many more people living minimally enjoyable lives.

The utilitarian focus on the efficient use of resources to maximize welfare outcomes has *prima facie* intuitive appeal. One of the biggest problems with public health, particularly in developing countries, is the inefficient use of resources. For example, many millions of rands of "irregular expenditure" (often representing corruption of one form or another) in healthcare are reported by South Africa's Auditor General every year. Historically, governments have sometimes paid more for basic medical supplies for their hospitals than an individual might pay in a pharmacy; tenders are often awarded to middlemen who outsource the work, taking a large chunk of the health budget in profit for doing nothing that benefits the public, and so on. Improving efficiency would make an enormous difference to the quality of healthcare. However, the utilitarian approach is clearly flawed. It fails to accommodate the egalitarian aspects of good public health policy.

5.3 Rawls's Theory of Justice

In order to circumvent the problems with the utilitarian approach concerning egalitarian issues, I (like others before me) believe one can draw inspiration from the principles Rawls sets out in his Theory of Justice. Norman Daniels, for example, suggests that the Rawlsian principle of "fair equality of opportunity" is more salient to public health policymaking, than the direct focus on welfare. Daniels highlights how without a certain degree of health, one cannot pursue the kinds of plans ordinary people within societies are likely to make; that is, to borrow from Daniels, being healthy (at least to some degree) is necessary for one to have a "normal opportunity range" (Daniels 2008, p. 43). Let us begin with Rawls's thought experiment: The Original Position.

In order to ground his social contract theory of justice in fairness and impartiality, Rawls sets up a thought experiment somewhat similar to Thomas Hobbes's 1651 "State of Nature" idea in *Leviathan*. He asks us to imagine a group of free and equal individuals gathered to deliberate over and establish a set of rules or principles of social and political justice for democratic societies. Unlike in *Leviathan*, Rawls stipulates that participants must be shrouded by the" veil of ignorance"; that is, they must not know their position in society. Whilst they *do* know basic economic principles, the desirability of basic social goods (and the consequences of their absence), laws of natural science, biology, psychology, and so on, they do not know where in the social hierarchy they sit, their wealth, their immutable properties such as race or sex, nor their religious or political commitments. Nor do they know their talents, skills, degree of education, or the history of the society in which they live. In this way, Rawls ensures that participants would not be able to tailor the principles of social justice to favour their individual circumstances, ultimately resulting in a maximally fair social contract.

Rawls presents the principles he believes would come from such deliberations. There is not space to critique the principles, here, but since they have (at least on the face of it, and at least in part) motivated a number of the ethical theories discussed later in this chapter, and that I personally find the values Rawls identifies intuitively appealing, I assume (perhaps foolishly) that they're agreeable enough to my reader. The principles relevant to public health (in the broad sense discussed in Chap. 1) are as follows:

1. *First Principle*: "Each person has an equal right to the most extensive total system of equal basic liberties compatible with a similar system of liberty for all." (Rawls 1971, p. 266)

   The basic rights and liberties are further specified. These include:

   Liberty of conscience and freedom of association, (Rawls 1971, pp. 33–35); freedom of thought and freedom of speech and expression (Rawls 1993, pp. 340–360); the integrity and freedom of the person and the right to hold personal property; equal rights of political participation and their fair value (Rawls 1971, pp. 36–37); and the rights and liberties protected by the rule of law (due process, freedom from arbitrary arrest, etc.). (Freeman 2023)
2. *Second Principle*: "Social and economic inequalities are to satisfy two conditions. First they must attach to offices and positions open to all under conditions of fair equality of opportunity; and second they must be to the greatest advantage of the least advantaged members of society [the difference principle]" consistent with the just savings principle. (Rawls 1993, p. 281; Rawls 2001, pp. 42–43; Rawls 1999, p. 266 in Freeman 2023).
3. "*Principles for individuals*, include (a) *the natural duties* to uphold justice, mutual respect, mutual aid, and not to injure or harm the innocent (Rawls 1999, p. 51); and (b) *the principle of fairness*, to do one's fair share in just or nearly just practices and institutions from which one accepts their benefits, (which grounds the principle of fidelity, to

keep one's promises and commitments." (Rawls 1999, p. 52 in Freeman 2023).

4. "*The Priority Principles*: the principles of justice are ranked in lexical order. (a) The priority of liberty requires that basic liberties can only be restricted to strengthen the system of liberties shared by all. (b) Fair equality of opportunity is lexically prior to the difference principle. (c) The second principle is prior to the principle of efficiency and maximizing the sum of advantages." (Rawls 1999, p. 266 in Freeman 2023)
5. *The General Conception of Justice:* "All social goods—liberty and opportunity, income and wealth, and the bases of self-respect, are to be distributed equally unless an unequal distribution of (Rawls 1971) any or all of these goods is to the advantage of the least favored." (Rawls 1971, p. 302 in Freeman 2023)

In addition to the above, Rawls advocates for the principle of fraternity (solidarity), where:

> ...fraternity is held to represent a certain equality of social esteem manifest in various public conventions and in the absence of manners of deference and servility. No doubt fraternity does imply these things, as well as a sense of civic friendship and social solidarity, but so understood it expresses no definite requirement... The difference principle, however, does seem to correspond to a natural meaning of fraternity: namely, to the idea of not wanting to have greater advantages unless this is to the benefit of others who are less well off. (Rawls 1999, p. 90)

Rawls's Theory of Justice is a general ethical theory, but with clear applications within public health. The three core themes emerging from the above principles are liberty, equality, and solidarity. Whilst on the face of it, liberty might not seem to play a dominant role in public health, to assume this would be a mistake.

Freedom of speech and political freedom have a significant impact on the capacities of the population at large. If one assumes the broad interpretation of the capacities approach detailed in Chap. 1, then all capacities (both of individuals and emergent capacities of populations) can in principle contribute to health. This includes freedom of speech, the capacity to own property, and the capacity to exercise rights of political participation. But even if one eschews this broader approach, and takes a more interventionist approach to population health, where the domain of population health is restricted to what affects the physiological and mental health of the population, then issues such as freedom of speech and freedom from arbitrary arrest still make a difference. There are countless examples of political activists who have been imprisoned or killed for criticizing their governments, and freedom of speech is no doubt a determinant of mental health. Nevertheless, the (in)equality-related principles (equality and solidarity) are very obviously linked to healthcare policy. Inequalities in healthcare are rife, and public health policy has a profound effect on this.

Freedom of movement is explicitly tied to the fair equality of opportunity principle. The COVID-19 pandemic highlighted how salient this principle can be in the context of public health, as lockdowns not only prevented international travel, but confined individuals to their homes for extensive periods of time. However, the emphasis on "fair" here can be used to justify such policies. So long as policies such as lockdown don't apply solely to the least advantaged groups (as anti-freedom of movement policies did during the apartheid era in South Africa), and so long as they are warranted by other principles, then lockdown need not be in tension with Rawls's Theory of Justice.

Resources relevant to healthcare, much like "liberty and opportunity, income and wealth, and the bases of self-respect", are social goods. According to Rawls's General Conception of Justice, all social goods must be distributed equally, unless unequal distribution of such goods is to the advantage of the worst off in society. The reality, of course, is that none of these social goods are distributed equally, and that it is difficult to establish a fair method for such distribution. Since I am not a genius economist with the solution to all of life's problems, I will not attempt to resolve this issue. Save to say, it seems to me that those who work harder for longer with higher skilled jobs, at least on the face of it, deserve to be paid more than those who work less hard for less time at more menial tasks (this assumes an idealized situation where the equality of opportunity principle is upheld—which it rarely, if ever, is).[1] If CEOs were not paid

[1] I acknowledge that Karl Marx would object to this, on the grounds that our abilities are to a large extent not earned.

more than their secretaries, it would be difficult to find competent CEOs willing to do the job, and companies employing thousands of people would fail, leaving many unemployed. Although the current degree of inequality of income between CEOs and the lowest paid employees is, in my opinion, enormously unjust, inequality of income can nonetheless be warranted, and consistent with the "fair" distribution principle. But what about healthcare resources? Can health inequalities be justified?

According to (at least my interpretation of) Rawls, inequality in healthcare resources could only be justified if they were to the advantage of the least favoured. Clearly, poor health in an individual, or the relatively poor health of one population in comparison to another, cannot be to their advantage. Inequalities in healthcare resources can be justified on Rawls's account, but only if better healthcare opportunities are made available to the least favoured. In reality, healthcare inequalities run in the opposite direction. The higher up the social/wealth hierarchy one is, the better the healthcare opportunities. The social determinants of health also operate in this way. It's relatively easy for a wealthy person with a car to access and purchase nutritious food. It's far harder for those living in disadvantaged areas. The quality of water and sanitation, of health-related education, and so on, are all higher for the upper echelons of society than for the poor. These are wrongs that need to be addressed.

The intuitively unpalatable, inegalitarian implications of utilitarian welfarist approaches to public health ethics seem to be ruled out by Rawls's principles of liberty, equality, and solidarity. To allocate a wildly disproportionate quantity of public health resources to those living in urban areas violates Rawls's general conception of justice. Again, he says "All social goods—liberty and opportunity, income and wealth, and the bases of self-respect, are to be distributed equally unless an unequal distribution of any or all of these goods is to the advantage of the least favored." (Rawls 1971, p. 301). Healthcare resources and opportunities are social goods. Unequal distribution in favour of those living in urban areas will typically not "advantage the least favored". The same principle would apply to any policy promoting unequal allocation of public resources in favour of the wealthy.

Thus, following Rawls (and other who have followed in his footsteps), I assume that a good theory of public health ethics must have the values of liberty, equality, and solidarity at its core.

5.4 Principlism and Public Health

In Chap. 6 I propose a development of Childress et al.'s principlist approach to public health ethics. Principlist approaches to public health, such as Childress et al.'s and Kass's (2001), find their foundations in biomedical ethics—from Beauchamp and Childress's (1994) principlism. To fully grasp the public health equivalents, it is worth briefly discussing its biomedical counterpart.

Unsurprisingly, when one applies a utilitarian framework to the traditional domain of bioethics, one encounters similar problems to those outlined in Sect. 5.2. Important aspects of ethical decision-making in medicine are ignored when one focuses simply on maximizing utility, be that measured in terms of maximizing pleasure/minimizing pain, extending life, or whatever metric one chooses. In clinical medicine, for example, autonomy is widely considered to be of paramount importance. A blood transfusion may be necessary to save a patient's life, but should that patient's religious beliefs lead them to refuse the transfusion, the patient's wishes should be respected. Similarly, matters of justice are ignored by the consequentialist framework. Suppose two patients require a liver transplant: one an alcoholic, 65-year-old, well-loved politician, who takes care of their constituency, and one a 14-year-old boy living in poverty. Utility may be maximized by choosing to extend the life of the politician by a few years, but justice demands that the otherwise healthy 14-year-old boy has a greater claim. To address these problems, Tom Beauchamp and James Childress introduced a bioethical framework known as Principlism. (Beauchamp and Childress 1994).

Principlism comprises four core principles:

1. Beneficence
2. Non-maleficence
3. Autonomy
4. Justice

The beneficence condition demands that medical practitioners attempt to maximize the "good" they can do for patient. The non-maleficence condition, which typically takes priority over beneficence, demands that medical practitioners avoid causing the patient harm, unless the harm is sufficiently outweighed by the benefits. The first two conditions are thus roughly equivalent to a utilitarian framework. The autonomy conditions states that the decisions of a patient of sound mind should always be respected. Finally, the justice condition demands policies that do not discriminate against the least advantaged, such that e.g. those in positions of power are no more entitled to treatment than anyone else. In line with Rawlsian principles, discrimination in favour of the least advantaged does not violate the justice principle.

This is a book on philosophy of public health, and whilst bioethical principles should be of consideration in public health ethics, it does not follow that Beauchamp and Childress's principles will serve as an adequate framework for public health. The agent of interest in biomedical ethics is the individual patient; in public health, populations take centre-stage. Biomedical ethics and public health ethics typically deal with different kinds of policy—patient-centric policies, and population-centric policies, respectively. But populations don't have autonomy, the people that comprise those populations do. That's not to say respect for autonomy does not matter for public health policymaking. When governments are considering e.g. vaccine mandates, the fact that this would likely undermine the autonomy of large numbers of people is a salient factor. But what an autonomy condition would mean for an ethical framework within the context of public health requires further examination.

With respect to beneficence and non-maleficence, it becomes unclear which group of people the cost-benefit analysis applies to. Adopting the account of health advocated in this book, beneficence amounts to increasing the relevant capacities of the population (*en masse*) and those that comprise it, and non-maleficence the avoidance of reducing those capacities—but whose capacities? The total population of a country is just one of the populations public health policy affects. These populations have subsets that are populations (complex systems) in themselves, just as the organ is as much a complex system as the organism. A policy that maximizes benefits and minimizes harms for the total population, might put some of these subset populations at particularly high risk. One might argue that this risk is ameliorated by the justice condition in the principlist framework. Perhaps the justice condition, appropriately reinterpreted in the context of populations, could not be satisfied in such a situation.

Since Beauchamp and Childress's principlism is targeted at bioethics, it is not within the scope of this chapter to examine the view in more detail, here. However, as noted previously, the general strategy of formulating principles to guide public health ethics has been adopted by various authors.

Kass argues that the ethical framework for public health should involve a six-step process. These steps makes passing reference to the principles of principlism, and are couched as "an analytic tool, designed to help public health professionals consider the ethics implications of proposed interventions, policy proposals, research initiatives, and programs" (Kass 2001, p. 1777). These steps are:

1. *To identify the programme's goals* (Kass 2001, p. 1777).

Kass takes these goals always to involve the reduction of morbidity or mortality. Whilst there may be proximate goals to public health interventions, such as educating the public, ultimately, she argues, the success of a public health program must be measured by its effect on identified morbidity and mortality rates.

> "Of course, other types of benefits, generally social benefits, can accrue from public health programs as well. Public health programs can result in greater employment, for example, as well as less tangible benefits, such as coalition-building or the strengthening of communities. These benefits are extremely important and should be given strong consideration. They are, however, the incidental or intermediary outcomes of public health programs, rather than the programs' final goal." (Kass 2001, p. 1778)

Kass is thus both operating within the narrow understanding of public health identified in Chap. 1. (that is, outcomes that pertain only to physiological/mental health—which is perfectly understandable, in context), and claiming that the goals of public health interventions concern only individual health outcomes. My account of the goals of public health concerns promoting both individual and population level capacities. Although improved individual health outcomes are an integral part of that, it seems to me that the *duty* of public health institutions is to provide opportunities to improve health (and remove/mitigate against obstructions to good health). To some extent, whether those opportunities are taken can be up to the individuals. To suggest otherwise, I think, can have important implications on liberty and autonomy.

2. *The effectiveness of the programme in achieving its stated goals.*

Kass argues that the likely effectiveness of the interventions must be established through evidence. Programmes are initiated through making certain "assumptions". Policymakers must identify what these assumptions are, and "what data exists to substantiate each of them" (Kass 2001, p. 1778). She highlights how the greater the burden posed by the programme on issues such as liberty and the economy, the better the evidence necessary for the programme's likely effectiveness. This is broadly in line with my own intuitions, and the principles of evidence-based public health noted in Chap. 3.

3. *Identify the "known or potential burdens of the program"* (Kass 2001, p. 1779).

Some public health interventions come with enormous burdens to populations. The almost global COVID-19 lockdown highlighted that. But ultimately, nearly all public health interventions entail some kind of a burden, economic or otherwise. These burdens need to be clearly identified in advance. Kass writes that "Whilst threats to autonomy are the most obvious threats posed by public health regulations and legislation, such regulations and legislation can, in some circumstances, be associated with physical risks, or risks to individuals' health, as well [e.g., federally approved and mandated vaccinations]" (Kass 2001, p. 1779). Public health interventions can also, she claims, pose a risk to the "justice" principle of principlism, should the burdens unfairly weigh on the disadvantaged. Little is said with respect to what burdens should be considered, and I will speak to this in Chap. 6.

4. *Identify how to minimize the burdens. Consider alternative approaches.*

Once step 3. is completed, public health policymakers have a duty to find ways to minimize these burdens, or find alternative strategies that achieve the same goals but with fewer burdens. We are ethically required, she argues, to "choose the approach that poses fewer risks to other moral claims, such as liberty, privacy, opportunity, and justice, assuming benefits are not significantly reduced" (Kass 2001, p. 1779).

5. *Implement the program fairly.*

Steps 5. of Kass's approach is consistent with Rawlsian distributive justice, and with the justice principle of principlism. It concerns "the fair distribution of benefits and burdens" (Kass 2001, p. 1780), such as access to clean water and access to preventative and curative medicine. Kass specifically mentions Daniels's (Daniels 2008) contribution in this regard, and his suggestion of "the need for all members of society to be brought to a level of "species-typical normal functioning"" (Kass 2001, p. 1781). I find this degree of distributive justice implausible, on the grounds that (a) it is impossible: it is physically impossible to bring the terminally ill and many disabled people to species-typical normal function, and (b) distributing resources in an attempt to do so would result in substantial "levelling-down". The cost burden of trying to bring (some of) the least healthy to species-typical normal function would be so high, that too many others would suffer. Whilst fair distribution of health resources will inevitably require an unequal distribution in favour of the least advantaged, the bar Kass sets (via Daniels) is too high. One needs to determine how unequal the distribution of health resources should be through a cost-benefit analysis.

6. *Identify how the "benefits and burdens of a program can be fairly balanced"* (Kass 2001, p. 1781).

Once the first five steps are completed, the final step is to determine whether and how the benefits and burdens of the intervention can be fairly balanced. Kass notes how there will inevitably be disagreements. People will disagree on the burden of banning smoking in public spaces, reporting one's name to the state, immunizing children, and so forth. Solutions to these disagreements, Kass argues, "must be reached through a system of fair procedures. Procedural justice requires a society to engage in a democratic process to determine which public health functions it wants its government to maintain, recognizing that some infringements on liberty and other burdens are unavoidable." (Kass 2001, p. 1781). In Chap. 6. I endorse a similar consultative process. Finally, Kass highlights how the "more uneven the benefits and burdens (that is, burdens are imposed on one group to protect the health of another), the greater must be the expected benefit" (Kass 2001, p. 1781). This, again, I consider to be a sensible principle.

In the formulation of her six steps, Kass draws on the principles of biomedical ethics. They bring justice, beneficence, non-maleficence and autonomy into the equation. The potential for conflict is noted, and she advocates for a democratic solution to this conflict to avoid the paternalist consequences of any alternative.

Kass's framework is broadly in line with Rawls's principles. It takes into consideration the effects of public health interventions on liberty and other social goods, as well as distributive justice. Although I disagree with Kass on the goals of public health, having argued in Chap. 2. that the goal of public health is to develop relevant capacities at both the individual and population scale, I agree that the goals of the intervention must be clearly identified in advance, and I broadly agree with the five steps that follow (save for the minor objections already noted). My main goal in Chap. 6. will be to provide greater specificity on the particular outcomes public health interventions should aim for, and the effects to avoid. But before moving on to that project, let me first discuss an alternative principlist approach: that of Childress et al.

Childress et al.'s General Moral Considerations

Whilst Childress et al. do not refer to their ethical tenets as principles, nor do they use the phrase "principlism" in their work, it's clear that what they provide is at least inspired by principlism in bioethics (Childress et al. 2002). First, because the four principles of principlism all appear among their "general moral considerations" for public health; second, because the general approach is much the same. Both the principles of principlism and the "general moral considerations" of this ethical guide to public health, are general rules applicable to health-related ethical decisions (that sometimes conflict with one another); and perhaps third, that James Childress, first author of this paper on public health ethics, is one of the founders of principlism in biomedical ethics. It is therefore, I suggest, reasonable to refer to Childress et al.'s framework for public health ethics as broadly principlist.

Childress et al. begin by examining the Institute of Medicine's 1988 definition of public health, which states that "public health is what we, as a society, do collectively to assure the conditions in which people can be healthy" (Childress et al. 2002, p. 170). They draw two key conclusions from this. First, that it highlights the need for "cooperative behaviour and relationships built on overlapping values and trust" (Childress et al. 2002, p. 170), and second that it suggests a "far-reaching agenda for public health that focuses attention not only on the medical needs of individuals, but on fundamental social conditions that affect population levels of morbidity and mortality" (Childress et al. 2002, p. 170). I am sympathetic to this interpretation. Despite Childress et al. specifically outlining a framework applicable to the United States of America, it nonetheless draws attention to the importance of the society's values, and of course that value-systems can differ (at least to an extent) from one population to the next. This is as true within the American context, as it is intercontinentally. Further, it places emphasis on social conditions that affect health, rather than on more narrowly defined medical interventions such as the treatment of existing conditions, or preventative medical interventions such as vaccines. This definition admits of the provision of clean water and sanitation, access to nutritious food, and so on, as legitimate public health interventions.

They go on to identify three senses of "public" with which public health is concerned. The first is the "numerical public", or the target population. They argue that the numerical public "reflects the utilitarian view that each individual counts as one and only one", and raises questions concerning weighing up the effects of interventions on "gains in life expectancy with gains in health-related quality of life" (Childress et al. 2002, p. 171). Contrary to the account (of health as an emergent property of populations) advocated in this book, Childress et al.'s approach takes the health of a population to be solely determined by the aggregate health of its constituent parts (the individuals).

The second notion of "public" highlighted is the "political public"—this is defined as what "we collectively do through government and public agency" (Childress et al. 2002, p. 171). Governments have a duty to promote the health of their populations without unnecessarily infringing on the individual rights of its people. Governments may, at times, feel the need to implement coercive measures. Examples include mandatory vaccinations for children attending public schools, or rare emergency measures such as imposing lockdown conditions during an epidemic. These decisions, they argue, "must rest on moral reasons that the public in whose name the policies are carried out could reasonably be expected to accept" (Childress et al. 2002, p. 171).

The third notion of "public" is the "communal public". This refers to those outside the scope of government with the power to implement public health interventions. Although these groups (outside the political public) have more freedom insofar "as they do not have to justify their actions to the political public", there are still moral constraints on what can be done. Childress et al. list "respect for autonomy, liberty, privacy and confidentiality, and transparency in declaring conflicts of interest" as key considerations (Childress et al. 2002, p. 171).

Whilst the majority of the burden falls on the political public to look after the interests of the numerical public, ideally, the principles guiding public health ethics would cover interventions driven by the communal public, too. The principles outlined by Childress et al., couched as "general moral considerations", are as follows:

- Producing benefits;
- Avoiding, preventing, and removing harms;
- Producing the maximal balance of benefits over harms and other costs (often called utility);
- Distributing benefits and burdens fairly (distributive justice) and ensuring public participation, including the participation of affected parties (procedural justice);
- Respecting autonomous choices and actions, including liberty of action;
- Protecting privacy and confidentiality;
- Keeping promises and commitments;
- Disclosing information as well as speaking honestly and truthfully (often grouped under transparency); and
- Building and maintaining trust. (Childress et al. 2002, pp. 171–172)

One can immediately see parallels with Beauchamp and Childress's principlism in bioethics; beneficence, non-maleficence, justice and autonomy all make an appearance. As with principlism, Childress et al.'s "general moral considerations" will often come into conflict when it comes to particular interventions. For example, a vaccine mandate or lockdown might (although not necessarily) help avoid health-related harms to a population, but that comes at the expense of liberty (in terms of freedom of movement) and autonomy. However, one can envisage scenarios where respecting autonomy or demanding consent from all citizens for a public health intervention would not be in the public interest. Similarly, focusing interventions on urban areas might produce the most benefits, but at the expense of those living in sparsely populated rural areas. Whilst "explicating the demands of justice in allocating public health resources and in setting priorities for public health policies, or in determining who they should target, remains among the most daunting challenges in public health ethics" (Childress et al. 2002, p. 172), strict adherence to the consequentialist principles would inevitably lead to violations of the justice condition.

Childress et al. note that although some advocate a lexical ordering for such principles to determine priority, it's likely that for any such orderings to be practicable, "tight or narrow specifications of the relevant general moral considerations" (Childress et al. 2002, p. 172) would be necessary to reduce conflicts. In short, determining the appropriate weightings of these principles in an epistemic vacuum is impossible since these are affected by both contextual conditions and the nature of the issue at hand. That said, conflict most commonly arises between those principles/moral considerations that further the traditional goal of public health—for Childress et al., to promote the health of the numerical public—and principles that protect other values such as liberty and autonomy. The authors offer five core concepts to help policymakers decide whether a public health intervention is warranted, despite its unintended negative effects in these regards. These are:

- Effectiveness
- Proportionality
- Necessity
- Least infringement
- Public justification (Childress et al. 2002)

Determining the effectiveness of the proposed intervention is important, since if an intervention is going to impact liberty or autonomy, there must be good reason for it: there must be a high probability that the intervention will improve and/or protect the health of the public.

The proportionality condition highlights the need for cost-benefit analyses for public health interventions. Infringements of liberty, autonomy, privacy etc. (let us call these "coercive policies") must be outweighed by the benefits of the intervention, if that intervention is to be warranted.[2]

---

[2] The Nuffield Intervention Ladder is worth considering, on this point (Nuffield Council on Bioethics 2007).

It is possible for an intervention to be both effective and satisfy the proportionality condition, and *unnecessary*. Such a situation would occur where some alternative, equally effective strategy that does not impose coercive policies on the population is available. Proponents of a coercive intervention must therefore "have a good faith belief, for which they give supportable reasons, that a coercive approach is necessary" (Childress et al. 2002, p. 173).

The least infringement condition is similar to the necessity condition. It states that where coercive policies are necessary, policymakers have a duty to implement the version that infringes these values to the least possible extent (Childress et al. 2002, p. 173).

Finally, the public justification condition asserts that where all four of the other conditions are met, public health institutions have a duty to explain and justify the restrictions on liberty, autonomy, privacy, and so forth. Moral reasons for the public health intervention need to be communicated to those affected (Childress et al. 2002, p. 173).

In my estimation, Childress et al.'s principles/ "general moral considerations" in combination with the five conditions noted above, provide a plausible initial framework for public health ethics, broadly consistent with Kass's six steps. The Rawlsian idea of respecting the basic rights and liberties of individuals is respected, and the authors rightly recognize the nuances of unique public health issues that make a generalizable lexical ordering/ranking of the principles they propose practically impossible.

Childress et al. do not claim that the approach they outline is complete. Nonetheless, it is worth highlighting that it is not. Without additional work, it would be extremely difficult to implement their strategy. They highlight the importance of producing benefits and reducing harms, but say little about what constitutes benefits and harms. They note difficulties in weighing up extensions of life expectancy against improving quality of life, but no general account is given. They suggest that by the health of the public, they mean the aggregate health of the individuals comprising that population, but do not specify what they mean by health. These are not serious deficiencies in the paper. It is a short paper entitled "Public Health Ethics: Mapping the Terrain", not "A Comprehensive Guide to Public Health Ethics and Policymaking". However, in the next section I discuss Sridhar Venkatapuram's capabilities approach to public health ethics as one possible way of understanding the benefits and harms of health policies, the concept of health itself, and of using capabilities as a guide to public health ethics. Since Kass's contribution highlights a stepwise process, through which something like the "general moral considerations" are to be applied (a process I am in large part happy with, except in the details), in Chap. 6 I draw on both Childress et al. and Venkatapuram to produce a more comprehensive, capacities-based principlism, to help iron out the details of Kass's process.

5.5 The Capabilities Approach

In his book *Health Justice: an argument from the capabilities approach*, Venkatapuram advances an account of health as "a vital or basic cluster of capabilities and functionings" (Venkantapuram 2013, p. 111) that draws on, but significantly develops ideas from Nussbaum and Nordenfelt. Like Nordenfelt, Venkatapuram ties an individual's health to their (cap)abilities, as opposed to e.g. the absence of disease in the Boorsean sense. Venkatapuram is critical of Nordenfelt, insofar as although he takes Nordenfelt's approach to be on the right track, Nordenfelt stopped short of explicitly stating what (cap)abilities were necessary to be healthy—a critical step, according to Venkatapuram, if the ethical framework is to be of practical use. Further, whilst Nordenfelt endorses a context-sensitive approach, whereby different abilities may be necessary in different contexts in order to be healthy, Venkatapuram goes on to provide a universally applicable set of criteria, whereby to be healthy is to have the "health capability". He draws the specific capabilities from Nussbaum's work on human dignity.

> "The capability to be healthy (CH) is a person's ability to achieve or exercise a cluster of basic capabilities and functionings, and each at a level that constitutes a life worthy of equal human dignity in the modern world. Making use of Nussbaum's theory of central human capabilities (CHCs), the CH can be usefully understood as a 'meta-capability' to achieve or exercise ten CHCs. These ten CHCs together make up a minimal concep-

> tion of a fully human life, and provide the bases for determining the decent social minimum of entitlements in the relevant parts of an individual's life". (Venkantapuram 2013, p. 143)

Nussbaum produced a list of capabilities necessary for living a life "worthy of equal human dignity". Venkatapuram argues that to be healthy is to instantiate the meta-capability to achieve (or exercise) Nussbaum's ten central capabilities. He thus creates an intimate tie between human dignity, or what it takes to "make up a minimal conception of a fully human life", and health. It's worth noting Nussbaum's capabilities, here, not least because human health itself appears as one of the salient capabilities. These are:

1. being able to live a normal length of lifespan;
2. having good health;
3. maintain bodily integrity;
4. being able to use senses, imagination and think;
5. having emotions and emotional attachments;
6. possess practical reason to form a conception of the good;
7. have social affiliations that are meaningful and respectful;
8. express concern for other species;
9. able to play; and
10. have control over one's material and political environment. (Nussbaum 2006)

Venkatapuram (reasonably) interprets the second capability, that of "having good health", to refer to health in the biomedical sense of "absence of disease". But since the WHO defines health as "a state of complete physical, mental and social well-being and not merely the absence of disease or infirmity" (WHO 2024), to suggest that there's more to health than the absence of disease should not be dismissed as incoherent—and of course, the idea that health is more than simply the absence of disease is consistent with the account advocated in this book. Since Nussbaum's capabilities include aspects of the biological, the psychological, and the social aspects of health noted by the WHO, one can see why Venkatapuram is drawn to this.

In short, Venkatapuram argues that to be healthy, is to be able to instantiate Nussbaum's ten capabilities. If one has the capability of "having emotions and emotional attachments", then obviously one is able to have that capability. However, one need not currently have that capability in order to be *able* to have it. One may be in a position to gain that capability through e.g., therapy, so long as one has access to the necessary resources. Hence the notion of health as a "meta-capability". As an account of health, this may sound counterintuitive. One can, at least intuitively, be pathologically malnourished, whilst having the capability to become nourished. I'll return to this issue via an objection from Michael Selgelid, shortly.

Nussbaum's capabilities—again, targeted at human dignity as opposed to human health—cover the Rawlsian ideals of liberty and the fair distribution of resources.[3] The reference to being able to live a "normal life span" highlights the latter, and "to have control over one's material and political environment", "to express concern for other species", and to be "able to play", the former.

Venkatapuram "[sees] health as a capability and [relies] on Nussbaum's theory for the content of the capability" (Venkantapuram 2013, p. 143). Drawing no distinction between the capability to be healthy and health itself may sound strange, but as an account of health in the public health ethics context, such a view might be useful. Public health service providers and policymakers have plenty of moral duties, and often (though not always) these must be limited to ensuring the public are able to be capable of X-ing (where X is some basic human need), as opposed to actively X-ing. For instance, a government should ensure all its citizens are able to be able to e.g. play sports, but it has no obligation to ensure that they are able to play sports (are skilled, practicing sportsmen). They must have access to training and facilities, but need not (and indeed should not) be forced to train.

Nussbaum's capabilities approach is ultimately an ethical framework. It's not merely a descriptive account of what it means to live a life worthy of human dignity—it is a prescriptive account of moral entitlements. For Venkatapuram, then, (reasonably assuming his acceptance of Nussbaums

[3] Consistency with Rawls may not be an explicit goal of Nussbaum or Venkatapuram, but since I am drawn to Rawls's conclusions, I deem this a virtue of the theory.

conditions for living a life worthy of human dignity) the meta-capability of health is not only something desirable, but a (complex) human right. Since public health agencies, dominated by governments, are responsible for promoting public health, Venkatapuram's approach entails they have a moral duty to ensure citizens are healthy (in his sense)—that they instantiate all aspects of the health meta-capability.

5.6 Critique of the Capabilities Approach to Human Health, and Responses

Selgelid provides a number of objections to Venkatapuram's view. He begins by highlighting how "many bioethicists consider [human dignity] to be a virtually meaningless and/or vacuous concept" (Selgelid 2016, p. 27). If dignity is indeed "notoriously hard to pin down" as Selgelid suggests, then defining health in terms of dignity is (he says) *a forteriori* problematic. A stronger, related, objection, concerns the apparent implication that for Venkatapuram, no unhealthy people live lives worthy of human dignity. I agree with Selgelid that the latter is counterintuitive, particularly since protecting the dignity of the sick is the explicit aim of many organisations. The not-for-profit organization, *Dignitas*, for example, is dedicated to "palliative care, suicide attempt prevention, advance health care planning and assisted dying" (Dignitas 2024). They have "To live with dignity. To die with dignity" as their slogan. On the face of it, this slogan would make little sense if Selgelid's interpretation of Venkatapuram were accurate (but it is not).

Whilst Venkatapuram has written an article addressing objections to his view, this particular critique was overlooked (Venkantapuram 2016). Nonetheless, there are at least two possible responses. First, Selgelid suggests that the link between dignity and health on the capabilities approach to health is one of identity. This is not the case. Assuming we take Nussbaum's ten capabilities to be together necessary and sufficient for living lives worthy of human dignity, the same does not apply to Venkatapuram's account of health. For him, to be healthy is to have the *ability to achieve or exercise* these capabilities—a meta-capability. That does not imply *having* those capabilities, as Nussbaum's account of dignity does. Thus, they are not identical. Second, even if we accept that many bioethicists see human dignity as a vague, ill-defined, vacuous concept, one could argue that Nussbaum resolves that. There is nothing vague or ill-defined about her ten capabilities, whether one agrees with them or not. Perhaps most importantly, though, at no point does Venkatapuram equate health with dignity. He is providing an account of health, not dignity. His view should only be criticized on grounds affecting it as an analysis of health.

Selgelid's second objection is that the bar for health is set too low. Nussbaum's idea is to articulate ten minimally sufficient capabilities for living a life worthy of human dignity, but Selgelid argues that "it is easy to imagine lots of prototypical cases of people who we would (and arguably should) consider unhealthy (e.g. with chronic illnesses or disabilities of various sorts) but nonetheless live more than minimally decent lives" (Selgelid 2016, p. 28). I find this objection, as stated, equally unconvincing—largely because Selgelid has pointed to an identity relation between health and dignity, and that is not Venkatapuram's intention. However, the "low-bar" objection might still hold weight, albeit not for the reasons Selgelid identifies.

The first three of Nussbaum's capabilities pertain to physical ailments. If those with chronic illnesses fail to meet Nussbaum's threshold, then, *contra* Selgelid, they fail to meet the minimum requirements for human dignity. This might be a reasonable objection to Nussbaum, for the reason Selgelid identifies, but it doesn't follow that it's a successful objection to Venkatapuram's capabilities approach to health. His view is that health is a meta-capability—being able to have Nussbaum's health capability is necessary for health, not having Nussbaum's health capability. One can be very sick, but nonetheless capable of recovery. Someone in this position would count as healthy on Venkatapuram's capabilities approach. This certainly conflicts with the lay conception of health, so from a descriptive perspective, the bar does indeed look to be too low. But one should note that Venkatapuram is not attempting a descriptive account of health. He is proposing a revolutionary one—an approach that views health in an entirely new way, where people are healthy if they have the capability to obtain Nussbaum's capabilities. Whilst I think Venkatapuram is on the right track with respect to public health ethics, I suspect this is nonetheless problematic as an account of health. I discuss this further in Chap. 6.

Third, Selgelid highlights the binary nature of Venkatapuram's account: one is either healthy, or not healthy. A healthy person is able to have all the capacities Nussbaum identifies, and an unhealthy person is not. But this presents a line-drawing problem, similar to that Peter Schwartz raises in his objection to Christopher Boorse's Biostatistical Theory (Schwartz 2007). To what extent must someone be able to play in order to satisfy capability 9? How healthy must one be (in the absence of pathology sense) to satisfy condition 2? Whilst this a problem for many accounts of health and disease in the philosophy literature, comparative accounts of health such as that of Schroeder (Schroeder 2013), and that I defend in Chap. 1. of this book, can overcome this difficulty. Of course, it's as much a problem for Nussbaum's account of dignity as it is for Venkatapuram's account of health. Is it really plausible to suggest that someone who falls just below the threshold for the capability to express one's concerns about other species, but easily meets the thresholds for all other capabilities, does not live a life minimally worthy of human dignity? Similarly, if one does not have the meta-capability to express one's concerns about other species (perhaps there's a law preventing this), but one has all other capabilities (or at least the meta-capabilities), then is one necessarily unhealthy? Nussbaum and Venkatapuram might both bite the bullet and argue in the affirmative, but this conclusion is at least questionable.

Fourth, Selgelid notes how Venkatapuram says "nothing specific" about how some of Nussbaum's capabilities are health-related. Whilst it is beyond the scope of this book to do the empirical research to justify this claim, I would imagine that were one to conduct a survey, few would accept that the capability "to express one's concerns for other species" is a health concern (Selgelid 2016, p. 30). It may be true that restrictions on freedom of speech (regarding concern for animals, or any other matter) have implications for dignity and wellbeing, but more needs to be said on how this relates to health if Venkatapuram has any intention of his health concept being consistent with ordinary language usage. That said, again it is worth noting that Venkatapuram's account is not descriptive, but prescriptive. It concerns how we *should* view health, not how we do. As it happens, it should be clear from Chap. 1. (and will be reiterated in Chap. 6.), that I agree with Venkatapuram that freedom of speech can (at least in principle) matter to health on the "broad interpretation".

Finally, Selgelid suggests there is confusion between talk of health as a functioning and health as a capability. To highlight this issue, he quotes the following passage:

> When *a wellbeing functioning* such as achieving internal immunity from a vaccine is not possible, then *agency functionings* become much more important in the protection of *health functionings* and indeed, all other capabilities…The causal components of conversion skills, physical environment, and social conditions are thought to be distal factors of *health functionings* that are outside the purview of health sector interventions…And the abilities to convert commodities into *health functionings* will also vary across individuals and over the life course. (Venkatapuram in Selgelid 2016, p. 31)

As Venkatapuram puts it, Selgelid accuses him of a kind of "capabilities fetishism" (Venkantapuram 2016), suggesting that, as Boorse and others like him propose, it is functionings rather than capabilities that matter for health. However, once one fully grasps the nature of capabilities this objection is unconvincing.

Functionings both confer capabilities, and are the manifestation of capabilities. In order to be able to express one's concern for other species, one needs certain functionings: to speak or to write—but this is in addition to living in the kind of social environments that permit freedom of speech. Similarly, in order to have Nussbaum's capability for good health, one needs a heart that functions with sufficient efficiency (note that a heart that functions with typical efficiency is a heart capable of functioning with typical efficiency)—but one also needs education on how to live a healthy lifestyle. The same applies to the health meta-capability. Certain functionings are necessary conditions of instantiating this meta-capability, but that's not to say it's the functionings that play the dominant role. Most of Nussbaum's capabilities require both functionings and environmental factors to be realized in order to be instantiated by an individual—that is why public health is so important for providing the health meta-capability. Good public health policy and proactive governance can ensure these social and environmental factors (institutions, laws, facilities) are in place.

5.7 Conclusion

In this chapter I showed that whilst welfarist utilitarian approaches are useful in some contexts (a utilitarian calculus will ultimately form a part of the ethical framework proposed in the next chapter), utilitarianism alone gives rise to undesirable consequences. Notably, that poorer rural communities and other vulnerable groups might be excluded from public health interventions due to their relative cost-per-capita.

Drawing on Rawls's Theory of Justice, I outlined the core principles a feasible and just public health ethics should respect; namely, the principles of liberty, equality and solidarity. Both Kass and Childress et al.'s principlist approaches deal with the issues faced by utilitarianism, and are consistent with Rawlsian ideals, but their accounts require further development. I engage in that project in the next chapter.

I ended the chapter with a discussion of Venkatapuram's health capability: a novel and intriguing approach to health. Whilst his account of health itself is, in my opinion, counterintuitive (it remains unclear to me how someone with symptomatic cancer could ever plausibly be considered healthy), and that further questions arise regarding why Nussbaum's ten capabilities are those most applicable to health, this kind of approach is worthy of further investigation. In Chap. 6 I develop some of Venkatapuram's ideas, and incorporate them into a capacities-based principlist ethical framework based on Childress et al.'s groundwork.

6

Towards a Capacities-Based Principlism

6.1 Introduction

In this chapter I present a new approach to public health ethics at two distinct, but related levels. First, I consider public health ethics at the level of duties towards those individuals comprising populations. This is the standard target, and the focus of the previous chapter, since most writers on this topic have deemed the notion of populations/the public as a "super-organism" implausible (something I deny, but prefer the term "complex system"). Second, I consider the possibility of ethical duties towards populations as complex systems.

In Sect. 6.2, I compare and contrast Venkantapuram's (2013) approach to health and public health ethics with my own. In Sect. 6.3 I propose Capacities-Based Principlism, a development of Childress et al.'s (2002) ethical framework for public health, that draws on Nussbaum (2006) and Venkatapuram. Central to this approach is the need for public health policymakers to focus on the equitable promotion of individuals' capacities to live maximally healthy (in the biomedical sense) lives, and their capacities to live maximally happy, meaningful lives. I apply these principles to the contentious issue of assisted dying.

B. Smart, *The Philosophy of Public Health*,
https://doi.org/10.1007/978-3-031-98804-2_6

Finally, in Sect. 6.4, I present a separate ethical framework for dealing with duties toward populations as complex systems. I argue that despite not having minds/experiencing pain etc., it is not implausible to suppose that such duties towards complex systems exist. I conclude with a further tentative list of capacities-based principles to capture these duties.

6.2 Venkatapuram's Capabilities Approach to Health Vs. the Capacities Approach

In the previous chapter I claimed that Venkatapuram's capabilities approach to public health ethics is promising, responding to a number of objections to his view. However, his ethical framework remains problematic in certain respects, and (in my opinion) it comes at the expense of an account of health that fails to align with our most basic intuitions about the concept. In this chapter I propose a tentative account of public health ethics based on the capacities account of health adopted in Chap. 1. This draws on Venkatapuram's ideas, but rejects his view of health as a meta-capability (Venkantapuram 2013, p. 143). My capacities approach to public health ethics proposes that public health policymakers have a duty to promote certain capacities, both at the level of those individuals comprising the population, and certain emergent capacities of the population as a whole.

Venkatapuram's account of health combined with the (traditional) goal of public health has the desirable consequence of making public health policymaking primarily concerned with giving people the ability to gain capacities/capabilities. Being immune to yellow fever, for example, might be considered part of Nussbaum's "having good health" capability (Nussbaum 2006). The immunized individual has the capability to remain healthy, even when exposed to yellow fever. However, arguably no public health institution has a duty to ensure everyone is vaccinated against yellow fever. That might infringe on the freedom of those who choose not to be vaccinated. Public health thus does not have a duty to ensure everyone has the capability to fight off yellow fever. That said, some public health institutions arguably *do* (at least where yellow fever is prevalent, and the vaccine is available) have the duty to ensure that everyone can access the vaccine, should they choose to: that is, the ability to gain the capability to fight off yellow fever—the meta-capability. Venkatapuram's approach therefore seems to identify, by and large, the right duties for those working in public health.

If the goal of public health is (at least in part) to improve the health of the population, and health is what Venkatapuram says it is, then we get the right kind of results; that is, results that give people the opportunity to improve their health and wellbeing, but are not forced to.[1] Nonetheless, the capabilities approach to health is, as an account of organism-health, highly counterintuitive. Somebody suffering from cancer, even when suffering from severe symptoms, would be considered healthy on Venkatapuram's view, so long as they have the meta-capability to be healthy; that is, so long as they are able to gain the capacity to be in good biological health (perhaps they have the opportunity to use life-saving treatment, but choose not to).

On the question of health, I differ from Venkatapuram in at least three ways. First, I do not take health to be a meta-capability, let alone the specific ability to have Nussbaum's ten capabilities for living lives worthy of human dignity. As explained in Chap. 1, I take health to be measured in terms of the capacities of complex systems, both at the level of the individual organism, and the population. The cancer patient's health is not determined by their ability to gain first order capabilities (a meta-capability), but by their capacities—what they can do. The cancer patient suffering from serious symptoms is in poor health relative to most people, insofar as their condition diminishes their capacities. Second, whilst capacities share something in common with capabilities (Nussbaum's capabilities are capacities to do or think certain things), my approach to health at the individual level does not restrict the capacities to Nussbaum's ten. Rather, the more health-relevant capacities an individual has, the healthier they are.[2] On my broad interpretation of health, the capacity to express *any* concern is likely to be just as relevant to health as Nussbaum's capacity to express concern for other species. Third, whilst Venkatapuram

[1] There are potential exceptions, such as justifiably vaccine mandates—I will return to this, later.

[2] What counts as a relevant capacity is to be determined by appropriate experts, in consultation with the public. See Chap. 1.

considers health at the population scale to be only the aggregate of individual health, the capacities approach highlights the importance of the (weakly) emergent capacities of populations as complex systems. No individual can provide universal healthcare, but a population as a complex system can. This capacity—having the hospitals and the skilled workers and the funding necessary to provide universal healthcare[3]—contributes to the health of the population as a complex system.

So much for our differences on what constitutes health, but what about public health ethics? Whilst I consider populations to be complex systems that can instantiate the health property, whether we have ethical duties towards a population in this sense is another matter. Populations do not have agency. They do not have autonomy. They do not suffer. Those who comprise those populations have agency, autonomy, and the capacity to suffer. Those working in public health certainly have duties to individuals, but whether they have duties to the complex system is more contentious. I discuss this possibility, shortly, concluding in the affirmative.

Venkatapuram's strategy is essentially to align the concept of health with an ethical theory, such that improving public health (the goal of public health) simultaneously serves to achieve ethical goals. My approach must differ somewhat, since whereas I agree that public health ethics should largely concern what Venkatapuram terms "meta-capabilities", health itself concerns first order capacities. Furthermore, given my acceptance that populations as complex systems can instantiate the health property, I suggest that public health policymakers have ethical duties at two levels: duties to the individuals comprising the population, and duties to the population as a complex system.

[3] Thaddeus Metz has suggested to me in private correspondence that this seems more like a "means" than a "capability". I accept that I may be deviating somewhat from ordinary usage, but on my view, to have the capability to X (I prefer "capacity") will frequently reduce to having the means to X. Broadly speaking, one (or a population) has the Capability/capacity to X in circumstances C when, if circumstances C arise, one (or a population) can X. Circumstances C might be a change of the law entitling everyone to adequate healthcare, and X its provision. The hospitals and the staff are what provide this capacity.

6.3 Capacities-Based Principlism: Duties to Individuals

Since the basic welfarist/utilitarian approach faces such substantive problems (such as ignoring egalitarian issues—see Chap. 5), and since, although the principlist approach put forward by Childress *et al* deals with these issues within the Rawlsian framework endorsed in Chap. 5, it remains somewhat vague, in this section I attempt to put some meat on the bones of principlism via the capacities approach to understanding health.

Whilst one should value pleasure and happiness, and disvalue pain and unhappiness, it seems to me that to focus on these things alone omits much of what is important to the human experience. This is one of the core problems with Mill's utilitarianism—utility is understood in such a way that much of what gives our lives meaning is ignored. Much of what endows people with dignity is ignored. Much of what motivates our actions is ignored. All these concepts have been explored in detail in alternative value theories, and the capacities approach to public health ethics attempts to capture at least some of this.

My approach is grounded by the Rawlsian principles of liberty, equality and solidarity (Rawls 1999). It is sometimes easy for those in living in the West to take liberty for granted. But for many South Africans (for example) during the Apartheid era in the mid-to-late twentieth Century, freedom was something worth dying for. Freedom from oppression, freedom to pursue one's goals, economic freedom, the freedom to live a healthy life, and the freedom to live with dignity were all denied to South Africa's indigenous population; in short, black people were denied the freedom to live a maximally meaningful life. To have the capacity to X is, at least in part, to be free to X. The concept of freedom is therefore implicitly embedded in the capacities account.

Equality and solidarity, too, can be viewed through the lens of capacities. Some capacities are social goods, and other social goods contribute towards capacities. Rawls notes "liberty and opportunity, income and wealth, and the bases of self-respect" specifically (Rawls 1971, p. 302 in Freeman 2023). According to the Rawlsian account I broadly endorse, social goods must be distributed equally unless unequal distribution advantages the least favoured. Bringing the Rawlsian principles and the capacities approach together, since e.g. disabled people typically have fewer capacities (are least favoured), the disproportionate distribution of social goods to the disabled should come out at warranted. I therefore propose the following, amended version of principlism in the public health context:

Capacities-Based Principlism

1. Maximally enhance/increase the capacities individuals require to live happy, meaningful lives, free from disorders, without excessively curtailing or removing (other) capacities individuals require to live happy, meaningful lives, free from disorders (welfare utilitarianism);
2. Distribute resources that contribute to health-related capacities fairly (equal distribution, unless unequal distribution advantages the least favored—distributive justice), ensuring public participation in decision-making processes, including the participation of affected parties (procedural justice);

And, although one may argue these should be considered subsidiary to or derivative from the above,[4] to:

1. Respect autonomous choices and actions, including liberty of action;
2. Protect privacy and confidentiality;
3. Keep promises and commitments;
4. Disclose information as well as speaking honestly and truthfully (often grouped under transparency); and
5. Build and maintain trust.

Let me now expand on the capacities noted above. As I have already suggested, public health has the duty to provide the opportunity for individuals to improve or maintain their physical health (vaccination programmes, access to primary care facilities, etc), but not always the duty to

[4] My thanks to Chris Wareham for this observation.

realize that improvement. That might unduly infringe on Childress *et al*'s principle of "respecting autonomous choices and actions, including liberty of action" (Childress et al. 2002, p. 171) (I discuss this in the context of morally permissible vaccine mandates in the section on conflicting principles, below). Thus, with respect to principle (i) above, and so far as possible, public health policymakers/workers have the duty:

1. To ensure, to the extent possible, that individuals have the capacity to maximally prevent and/or cure physical and mental disorders.

This capacity is complex, involving a wide variety of stakeholders providing a wide variety of sub-capacities. Let us take a sub-capacity to be a capacity necessary for a further capacity. In this case, capacity 1. requires the population to have the sub-capacities to access health information and healthcare services. It means they must have the capacity to access clean water, good sanitation, vaccinations, adequate nutrition, and so on.

I say "to the extent possible", and "maximally prevent and/or cure", instead of "prevent and/or cure", since there are limitations on medicine and public health. Prevention or cure can be impossible, either in practice or in principle. Many people are born with incurable physical disabilities, incurable mental disorders, and so forth; many people develop chronic conditions in later life that could not have been prevented, and furthermore, the realities of health economics typically do not enable perfection. Yes, it makes sense for a disproportionate quantity of social good to benefit the least advantaged, but not all resources can be directed to the least advantaged. This would result in an overall reduction in population health as understood in Chap. 1. However, everyone can have the capacity to "maximally prevent and/or cure disorders" *given their unique physical/mental circumstances* "to the extent possible", should the right social circumstances materialize. Promoting capacities directly related to physical and mental health is likely the capacity most people expect public health to focus on, so the above should be relatively uncontroversial.

My analysis of health does not stop with addressing physical and mental disorders, however. Avoiding disorders endows individuals with all kinds of capacities, but those are not the only capacities of importance. Following Nordenfelt, I argued in Chap. 1 that the capacities contributing to health (at all levels of complexity) are those that contribute to the organism/organisms' "vital goals". Nordenfelt defines vital goals as "goals that are inherent in all humans…. The vital goals include survival but they encompass much more… A person's vital goals are, for Nordenfelt, the states of affairs that are necessary and jointly sufficient for his or her minimal long-term happiness. (Nordenfelt 2018, p. 14). Whilst I think Nordenfelt has the right kind of approach, I suggest we need to look beyond "happiness" and include "meaning in life" in our analysis.

One can be in good physical health, but unable to live a meaningful life. A population in good physical health but lacking the capacities necessary for meaningful lives is,at least arguably, not a fully healthy population—or, at least, is less healthy than those populations both in good physical health *and* living meaningful lives. Even if public health workers don't explicitly provide interventions pertaining to education, fiscal policy, and so forth (all of which affect health in the sense proposed by this book), those guiding macro public health policy are often (to an extent) the same people guiding social and economic policy—generally speaking, this is government. Decisions that affect education and fiscal policy, affect people's ability to live in good health—they are thus, in a very real sense, public health decisions. Public health policymakers in government therefore also have a duty:

2. To ensure, to the extent possible, that individuals have the capacity to achieve their vital goals: to live maximally meaningful, happy, pain-free lives.

Again, this is complex capacity, comprising many sub-capacities. I will not dwell on the notions of happiness and pain—the reader's intuitive understanding of both will suffice for my purposes. However, I will discuss why, unlike the utilitarian, I do not rely solely on happiness, but invoke both the capacity to prevent/cure disorders and the capacity to live meaningful lives.

Public health is in the business of improving the health of populations—however that is to be interpreted. Studies on happiness, taken as a measure of subjective wellbeing, have shown that people's levels of happiness are less correlated with health and wealth as one might think. For example, Strotmann and Volkert conducted a study in several villages in Karnataka, India. In the villages studied, 76.4% of the households studied were multidimensionally poor. (Strotmann and Volkert 2018). Multidimensional poverty considers three main dimensions: education, health, and standard of living, and the bar is low (Alkire and Foster 2011). Despite this, 85.6% of Strotmann and Volkert's respondents reported being either "happy", "fairly happy", or "extremely happy". One's subjective level of wellbeing is affected by many factors. Amartya Sen notes, for example, the importance of "what a person is free to do and achieve in pursuit of whatever goals or values he or she regards as important." (Sen 1985, p. 206), and with respect to health, that the "…internal view of the patient may be seriously limited by his or her knowledge and social experience. A person reared in a community with great many diseases and little medical facilities may be inclined to take certain symptoms as "normal" when they are clinically preventable" (Sen 2009, pp. 285–286).

That said, Branchflower and Oswald summarise the findings of the literature on happiness as follows:

> [Happy people are] disproportionally the young and old (not middle-aged), rich, educated, married, in work, healthy, exercise-takers, with high fruit-and-vegetables diets, and slim. […] Happy countries are disproportionally rich, educated, democratic, trusting, and [show] low-unemployment. (Branchflower and Oswald 2011; Strotmann and Volkert 2018, p. 172)

The Branchflower and Oswald paper reviews many international studies on happiness. It finds that happiness and low levels of poverty are correlated. But the Strotmann and Volkert paper highlights that high levels of subjective well-being can be experienced even in regions with high multidimensional poverty. So, whilst I am happy to accept happiness as a social good and something worth promoting, I think it reasonable to assume that focusing purely on happiness is unlikely to be optimal in public health ethics.

I say more on "meaning" in the next section, but for now it's worth noting that the specifics for what it means to live a maximally meaningful life can differ from one person to the next. For some, to live a maximally meaningful life may simply be to raise a family in safety and in good health. For others, it may involve social migration, buying a home, the ability to exercise freedom of expression, to be involved in politics, to become a health professional, to write books, or travel. This could never be an exhaustive list, but the key point is that people must have the freedom to pursue their goals—the things they (reasonably) love. The ability to live a meaningful life is essential to human wellbeing, and since according to the WHO, "Health is a state of complete physical, mental and social well-being and not merely the absence of disease or infirmity" (WHO 2024), the idea that the above is intrinsically tied to health should again not be dismissed as implausible.[5]

This book is not devoted entirely to public health ethics, and it is beyond its scope to develop or defend a particular view of human dignity, or indeed to discuss the idea in sufficient detail to do it justice. That said, I am certainly less sceptical of the notion than Selgelid (see Chap. 5). It seems to me that whatever human dignity is, we have a moral duty to promote dignified lives.

Nussbaum's capabilities approach to human dignity captures some of the sub-capacities necessary for living meaningful lives. For example, she explicitly refers to "meaningfulness" in capability 7: "to have social affiliations that are meaningful and respectful". I find Nussbaum's capabilities inadequate in certain respects. I accept that the ability to "express concern for other species" is important, but consider it no more important than the ability to exercise one's freedom of speech more generally (with the usual caveat of avoiding hate speech). That said, Nussbaum herself does not assert her list to be complete, and I will leave the reader to consider additional options.

Since Nussbaum's capabilities approach seems a *prima facie* plausible approach to human dignity, that the ability to live a meaningful life is a plausible condition for living with human dignity, and that ensuring

[5] See section "Potential objection: Health and Wellbeing are Different", below.

people live lives worthy of human dignity is a plausible moral duty, then promoting the capacity to live meaningful lives is a plausible moral duty.

6.4 The Meaning of Meaning

Meaning in life[6] can no doubt be understood in myriad ways, and I shan't claim that the version advanced here is the only plausible one. However, I draw on two prominent scholars in the area whose views are in broad agreement, and satisfy the needs of my proposal. Thaddeus Metz (2021) and Susan Wolf (2010) both begin by distinguishing the value of "meaning" from other notable values—specifically, "happiness" and "moral value". The general thought is that whilst adding meaning to one's life is a reason for action, what is meaningful need not promote happiness, nor need meaningful actions be morally praiseworthy. Wolf notes that staying up all night to sew a Halloween costume for one's daughter does not promote happiness. Nor does one do it out of a sense of duty. Rather, she argues, one completes such arduous tasks out of love (Wolf 2010, p. 4). Metz notes that whilst cultivating a garden or mastering chess may be neither pleasurable nor morally praiseworthy, these are nonetheless activities that many are driven to perform. Why would we be so inclined, given the backbreaking nature of gardening and the lack of a duty to do these things? The answer, it seems, is that there is another form of value: "meaningfulness". One cannot, however, define a value solely through what it is not.

To address this, Metz suggests that meaning can be viewed as a cluster of properties:

[6] A brief complaint: I don't like the use of the word "meaning" to convey the value the literature on "meaning in life" attempts to convey. Traditionally, "meaningful" is a predicate applicable to language. For a word to be meaningful is for it to refer. For Wittgenstein, "meaning is use" (Wittgenstein 2009); what a word means is determined by how that word is used by ordinary language users in various language games. None of this is remotely related to the new usage of "meaningful", which has taken on a meaning of its own. That said, since meaning is use, and since and there is a growing body of literature on meaning in life (and indeed, ordinary language users will now sometimes complain about a lack of meaning in their lives), here I attempt explain what the new (additional) meaning of meaning is meant to be.

> Thinking about meaning in a life may be taken to involve a non-instrumental value in a person's life, i.e., something that makes her life more desirable apart from other goods it might bring about, that comes in degrees and involves things such as achieving a higher purpose, relating positively to value beyond oneself, meriting pride, making sense, making a contribution, and being the author of a life. (Metz 2021, p. 444)

Wolf suggests that meaningfulness is "a category of value that is not reducible to happiness or morality, and that is realized by loving objects worthy of love and engaging with them in a positive way" (Wolf 2010, p. 13). Wolf's account of "meaning" amounts to two individually necessary and together sufficient conditions. First, loving objects worthy of love. Loving objects *simpliciter* is insufficient since one may love many things not worthy of love, and these cannot lead to enhancing meaning in life. One might love gambling or drugs, but neither promote meaning. Wolf describes this as involving both a subjective and an objective component. The agent must "care fairly deeply about something… as opposed to being bored or alienated from all that she does", but this thing/person/activity must have "objective attractiveness". Due to space constraints I will not attempt to outline conditions for "objectively attractive",[7] but assume the reader will have some intuitive notion of the kinds of thing that count: family and friends, intellectual pursuits, charity, art, music, literature, and so on.

Second, "engaging with them in a positive way". It is not enough simply to love objects/people/activities etc., one needs to be able to engage with them in a way that's supportive or constructive. One needs to be able to tend to one's family and friends, play musical instruments, read the literature, and write the philosophy. Of course, one need not do all, or indeed any of these specific things to live a meaningful life, but positive engagement with worthwhile "objects" one cares deeply about is, for Wolf, the essence of a meaningful existence. For the purpose of this

[7] Indeed, Wolf fails to describe such conditions. She does, however, have this to say: "When we consider what deep human interests or needs a meaningful life distinctively answers to… the objective aspect of such a life needs to be stressed. Our interest in living a meaningful life is not an interest in a life *feeling* a certain way, but rather an interest that it *be* a certain way, specifically, that it be one that can be appropriately appreciated, admired, or valued by others" (Wolf 2010, p. 32)

book, and since Wolf's account seems largely consistent with Metz's,[8] I am happy to endorse Wolf's characterization of "meaning".

6.5 The Capacity to Live Happy, Meaningful Lives, Free of Disorder

I argued in Chap. 1 that health should be measured through capacities, both at the individual and population levels. Furthermore, in Chap. 2 that the proper goal of public health is to increase these capacities—particularly those population-level capacities that provide opportunities for individuals to improve their health. Some of these capacities can lead to additional happiness (in individuals), some of them to additional meaning, and some of them to both. Beyond providing individuals with the capacity to live lives (maximally) free from physical and mental disorders, I have claimed that the core duty of public health is to provide people with the capacity to live meaningful lives.

The principlist approach I suggest has its benefits over standard utilitarianism. As I have already suggested, improving the physical health of the most advantaged might well have a greater positive impact on net happiness than improving the health of someone (of the same age) living in extreme poverty. Privileged people are likely to live longer. The utilitarian approach, therefore, seems to promote focusing public health interventions on the privileged. Capacities-based principlism asks that resources that promote capacities (including those required for enhancing both meaning and happiness) are equally distributed, *unless to the advantage of the least favoured.*

It is likely also true that privileged people are able to lead meaningful lives in more ways than underprivileged people. They are typically better

[8] Note that Metz does not think one must be attracted to the objectively worthwhile activities, but accepts that often more meaning accrues if one is. He further attempts to specify the worthwhile activities, viz., in terms of positive exercises of intelligence (Metz 2013).

educated and better able to read, write, and produce art. They are more able to engage in charity work, and so on. However, meaningfulness can be obtained in many ways, some of which do not require much wealth, and the number of ways in which people are able to obtain meaning is less important than the degree of meaning that can be obtained. People raise children in the most difficult of circumstances, they can play an active role in improving their communities, and so on.

Policymakers should thus not consider only their policies' effects on physical/mental health, but also their effects on other capacities. These include the capacity to read. Thus, the dual duties to (i) provide all with the capacity to live maximally meaningful, happy lives (ii) maximally free of physical/mental disorders, does not disadvantage the poor in the way a duty to maximize happiness in the population might.

So, what kind of interventions are to be prioritized in order to give everyone the capacity to lead meaningful lives free of disorders? I cannot answer this question in full, here. However, I tentatively suggest the below are of particular importance. These capacities enable one to pursue many of the meaningful activities noted above, from reading to caring for loved ones to raising children in safety. Whilst not all these capacities are in the traditional purview of the profession of public health, each contributes to the wellbeing of those comprising populations, and to health as I define it. Accordingly, public health policymakers should bear any effects on these capacities in mind when making policy decisions.

1. The capacity to access safe, affordable housing;
2. The capacity to access electricity;
3. The capacity to access clean, running water and sanitation;
4. The capacity to access employment (when necessary, with equal opportunities, and adequate pay);
5. The capacity to access affordable, nutritious food;
6. The capacity to access quality education;
7. The capacity to access quality preventative and curative medical interventions;
8. The capacity to freely express oneself without fear of consequences (excluding hate speech);

9. The capacity to make autonomous choices (that do not infringe on the rights of others);
10. The capacity to be politically active (e.g. to protest, to vote, to be elected);
11. The capacity to move freely, and safely, at least within one's own country;
12. The capacity to live (maximally) free of crime and/or the fear of crime;
13. The capacity to live (maximally) free from discrimination (racial/sexual/gender, etc.);
14. The capacity to form loving relationships.
15. The capacity to play.
16. The capacity to enjoy aesthetics (participate in the arts, be a spectator of the arts/sports, access natural beauty, etc.)

The sixteen capacities noted above are not exhaustive, but the promotion of each are important to health, and each promotes the Rawlsian values of liberty, equality and solidarity. Liberty insofar as freedom of speech and autonomy and the capacity to be politically active are essential to freedom, and equality and solidarity insofar as these are capacities policymakers have a duty to ensure all enjoy, and not some at the expense of others. Again, they should be distributed fairly, and where there is an unequal distribution, it should benefit the least advantaged. It is arguable, for example with respect to capacity 13, that historically oppressed groups should be afforded greater protection against e.g. racial or gender discrimination than historically advantaged groups. The same principle applies to the other capacities.

Of course, public health institutions are not responsible for promoting many of these capacities. The point is that public health institutions should consider, in their evaluation of the impact of their interventions, the effect of the intervention on each of these capacities; and further, that any institution "doing something" that affects one of these capacities, is having an effect on the health of the population.

6.6 Assisted Dying: A Case Study

The ethics of public health and biomedical ethics are distinct, but often related fields. The ethics of voluntary euthanasia, or assisted dying, is one such situation. The decision of a doctor to help a patient terminate their life is a matter for biomedical ethics. The legalization of assisted dying is (at least arguably) a public health policy decision made by lawmakers. It involves vulnerable population protection, and has healthcare system implications. In this section, I briefly consider what the capacities approach to public health ethics would suggest concerning the question of legalizing voluntary euthanasia.

I have suggested endorsing a broadly principlist approach to public health ethics, with a focus on promoting certain capacities. Specifically, maximizing the capacity to live free from physical and mental disorders, and maximizing the capacity to live meaningful, happy, pain-free lives. Terminating life, whether before it has properly began in the case of abortion, or sometime in adulthood, terminates the capacity to live meaningful happy lives free from pain and disorder. At a cursory glance, the capacities-based principlist approach would look unfavourably on voluntary euthanasia. However, a less superficial investigation suggests a more nuanced conclusion.

Capacities-based principlism asks that we "respect autonomous choices and actions, including liberty of action". Voluntary euthanasia, by definition, involves respecting the autonomous choice of the patient to end their own life. In cases where patients not only lack Nussbaum's capabilities necessary to live a life worthy of human dignity, but also lack the meta-capability to have these capabilities at any point in the future, it's arguable that terminating the patient's life is causing them little harm, and in fact alleviates suffering. In these circumstances, and to the extent possible, doctors should strive to respect patient autonomy (Beauchamp and Childress 1994), and public health should create an environment where doing so is legal.

But what of the seemingly conflicting principles of enhancing capacities to live meaningful, happy, pain-free lives? Ending the life of a patient necessarily ends the possibility of them living a meaningful life or experiencing any further happiness. The obvious response is that those looking to end their lives are in the best position to judge the quality of their lives—whether they are living lives worthy of human dignity. No physician can experience the pain a patient is in. No physician can tell a patient how meaningful their lives are. They do not have first person privilege. Ultimately, the patient is the person best positioned to make these judgements.

A doctor can and should inform a patient in pain whether their physical situation is likely to improve. Most cases of assisted dying, however, concern either patients with terminal illness, or patients with chronic conditions with little chance of significant improvement. If a patient is living with chronic pain, where painkillers are not enough to help the patient live a life worth living, there is a very real sense in which ending the life can be the best course of action to minimize the pain. Similarly, if, after due consideration, a paraplegic patient believes their lives lack any meaning—that they are incapable engaging with objects worthy of love in a positive way—then extending their lives is not going to increase meaning. Furthermore, ending their life is not going to diminish their capacity to live a meaningful life, since by their own estimation, their life is devoid of meaning.

Using the idea of "narrative meaning", having a dignified "ending" to one's life might make the completed life more meaningful (Singer 2004). There is little a doctor can do to enhance the capacities of the individual required to live a happy, meaningful life, free from disorders; and ending their life does not prevent or remove the capacities of the individual required to live a happy, meaningful life, free from disorders. Since their condition is *ex hypothesi* incurable, there is little risk of getting this wrong. Finally, on the assumption that the patient is right in their assessment of the quality of their life, and that the doctor is right in their assessment of the probability of improvement (and I take it these are assumptions we should make, unless we have good reason not to), then ending the patient's life likely respects principle of producing the maximal balance of increasing and decreasing relevant capacities. It would eliminate the capacity of the patient to experience physical or emotional pain.

It is worth noting that the extent to which pain is reduced by voluntary euthanasia is in fact increased relative to terminal illness in cases of non-terminal but chronic illness, and thus (in contrast to much legislation where assisted dying is legalized) having a terminal illness should not, in my opinion, be a precondition for legal voluntary euthanasia. In short, capacities-based principlism supports lawmakers enabling assisted dying, at a minimum in circumstances such as those described above.

6.7 Potential Objection: Health and Wellbeing are Different

Including the promotion of happiness and "meaning in life" in one's account of health makes wellbeing a central aspect of the concept. But the WHO definition of health, which explicitly highlights the inclusion of wellbeing in addition to living disorder-free, has come under fire. For those who feel a sharp distinction should be drawn between wellbeing and health, the account presented above will be unconvincing. Daniel Hausman, for example, states that the WHO definition conflates "health and wellbeing, and although it has never been formally repudiated, the World Health Organization does not rely on this definition in its attempts to measure health" (Hausman 2015, p. 18; Valles 2018). However, I agree with Sean Valles (2018) that those criticizing the WHO's account are misguided. The problem with this kind of objection, Valles notes, is that "departures from "normal functioning" only represent some of the ways that health can be harmed" (Valles 2018, p. 64). Health can also be harmed through e.g., spiritual harms and identity harms (Valles 2018, p. 64).

Even if health is currently measured by reference to normal biological function alone, it does not follow that this is the best way to measure the health of individuals or (through aggregation) of populations. In Chap. 1. I offered a prescriptive account, not a descriptive one. My capacities account of health takes the idea that health is purely the absence of disorder to be mistaken. Health should be a richer notion than that, more in line with the WHO definition—which, as Hausman himself notes, remains unrepudiated. Valles goes on to argue that:

> Critics have mistaken what the WHO definition is and does: it outlines a meta-concept of health, a conceptual frame-work within which particular operational concepts of health can be specified for particular purposes in particular communities—the WHO definition is not an operational definition to be used in applied research or policy "off the shelf… the question is not whether the WHO definition is the right *tool* for doing population health work; the question is whether the WHO definition is the right sort of *toolbox* for collecting tools for doing population health work. (Valles 2018, pp. 65–66)

This claim is later substantiated by example. The WHO *do*, as a matter of fact, develop tools using this toolbox. Valles highlights this through the UN-WHO programme "Every Woman. Every Child.", which "uses a life course model… to conceptualize the well-being of women as being practically inseparable from the health of children and adolescents due to the global prevalence of social and biological bonds through birth, childcare, etc" (Valles 2018, p. 67).

Some might remain unconvinced by this. They might argue, for example, that whilst the "Every Woman. Every Child." project indeed shows that the WHO acknowledge a relationship between wellbeing and health, wellbeing is viewed as a determinant of health, not an aspect of it. Perhaps that is true—but if so, it makes little difference from a policy perspective. Whether wellbeing is considered an important determinant of health, or an aspect of health itself, wellbeing is something public health institutions and policymakers need to pay attention to, and in many instances, act on.

Valles defends a "life course" theory of health. For him, health (1) should not be assessed at a single moment in time, and "must be assessed with respect to a developmental trajectory that occurs over time", and that "individuals' health develops through dynamic relationships with the healths of their population and their social-environmental contexts" (Valles 2018, p. 59). Whilst I fully agree with (2), I'm not so convinced that health cannot be measured at a single moment in time. My capacities account of health is forward looking, insofar as what matters is what the individual/population can do (now and at future times). Nonetheless, the approach I endorse allows one to be in relatively good health one moment, then contract a virus and be less healthy the next.

Of course, it does not follow that public health institutions are responsible for *all* interventions relevant to health, in this broad sense. Improving the health of populations requires growing economies, developing the education system, ensuring an adequate justice system and welfare state, as well as the traditional role of public health. Public health institutions must restrict their interventions to those that develop the capacities on the narrow (physiological/mental health) interpretation of health (Chap. 1). After all, they are not equipped to do anything else. But all major spheres of government contribute to the happiness and meaningfulness of peoples' lives—their health—and it is vitally important that public health does not operate in a vacuum. Interventions with a negative impact on the economy disproportionate to the benefits for (physical) health should not be implemented, and governments must ensure that systems are in place to prevent that from happening. Public health policymakers must therefore work together with experts from other fields (education, economics, etc) so they can properly assess the overall impact of their interventions, and make informed decisions.

Both Childress *et al* and Venkatapuram consider public health ethics to concern the effects of public health policy on individuals. The section above on capacities-based principlism does the same. For Venkatapuram and Childress *et al*, this is unsurprising, since the health of populations (or "the public") is, for them, at most a metaphorical notion capturing the aggregated health states of those comprising the population. I have argued in this book, however, that at least some populations are complex systems instantiating weakly emergent properties, and that health is one of these properties. Specifically, populations that satisfy the criteria outlined in Chap. 1: nonlinearity, feedback loops, self-organization and adaptation—these are applicable to e.g., societies, rather than "the human race" *en masse*. The question arises, then, whether in addition to having duties to those comprising these populations, public health policymakers have duties to populations as complex systems. I argue that they do.

6.8 Motivating Duties towards Populations as Complex Systems

Populations as complex systems do not experience pleasure or pain. They do not live meaningful lives in the sense of "meaningful" described above, since they cannot engage with objects of love in a positive way. Populations do not have minds. Capacities-based principlism as applied to individuals thus cannot be applied to populations as complex systems. However, my primary guide to ethical principles is intuition (my own, alongside my impression of the intuitions of others).[9] To illustrate why I think it's plausible to suggest we have duties to populations, consider similar arguments found in the environmental ethical literature.

Aldo Leopold (1949) has argued that "land is a community is the basic concept of ecology, but that land is to be loved and respected is an extension of ethics (Leopold 1949, pp. vii–ix)… A thing is right when it tends to preserve the integrity, stability, and beauty of the biotic community. It is wrong when it tends otherwise" (Leopold 1949, pp. 224–5).

Following Leopold, Holmes Rolsten III argues that we have a moral duty to protect species. It is highly counterintuitive, for example, to think it morally permissible to eliminate an entire species of e.g. a non-sentient insect, in order to increase the value of the specimens one has collected. Rolsten argues that species are "intrinsically valuable and are usually more valuable than individual specimens, since the loss of a species is a loss of genetic possibilities and the deliberate destruction of a species would show disrespect for the very biological processes which make possible the emergence of individual living things" (Brennan 2021).

Neither land, ecosystems, nor species are sentient things. In the case of non-sentient insects (assuming there are such things), neither the individual insects nor the complex system of the population of insects (in

[9] This strategy is not uncommon. Ethical theories are regularly criticized by appeal to their counterintuitive implications.

cases where these insects make up a genuine complex system—e.g. a bee hive), are sentient. They nonetheless seem to have inherent value. If the intuition is that it is wrong to eliminate these populations is correct—an intuition that I share—then, assuming we are also willing to assign value to human populations, we have duties to human populations *qua* complex systems, just as we do to the individuals that comprise these populations.

Suppose a small, isolated, African people (or clan) is facing a health crisis, and that this clan satisfies the conditions for being a complex system. Further, suppose that the country's public health authority has the option of either allocating funding to deal with that crisis, rescuing the clan from likely extinction, or allocating it to improve healthcare in suburbia, where the funds would likely save a few more lives/improve the physiological health of a few more people. Where should the funding go?

I suggest that we typically value the continued survival of African peoples. That whilst individual deaths are *ceteris paribus* equally regrettable, we would typically disvalue the eradication of an entire culture embodied in that complex system, more than we would disvalue a similar number of deaths among a much larger population that would persist despite those deaths. The fact that we value the survival of cultures and populations, and on the assumption that the moral duties we (at least think we) have ultimately derive from these values, is sufficient to provide a *prima facie* case for moral duties towards at least some populations as complex systems.

6.9 Population-Level Capacities-Based Principlism

As mentioned, the capacities-based principlism previously set out cannot work at the level of populations, since populations do not have experiences such as happiness. However, as I have already argued, they do have capacities, and whilst a population does not have a mind, there is a metaphorical sense in which it has agency, exemplified through democracy. I therefore propose a further broadly principlist ethical framework at the population-level. This involves promoting the (emergent) capacities of populations as complex systems. Ultimately, this amounts to promoting the health of populations (as complex systems) as described in Chaps. 1 and 2. The duty of public health policymakers and workers with respect to populations by and large align with achieving its goal. Whilst I do not take this to necessarily be an exhaustive list, public health policymakers should strive to:

1. Promote the capacities necessary for the continued survival and flourishing of populations as complex systems.
2. Promote the capacities necessary for the preservation of the cultural heritage of populations as complex systems (should this be "the collective will of the people").
3. Promote the capacities necessary for the positive development (technological, infrastructural, etc.) of populations as complex systems.
4. Promote the capacities necessary for the collective will (in the democratic sense) of populations as complex systems to be respected (where this does not violate the rights of individuals).

If this system were adopted, these principles would ensure that in the thought experiment above, the public health authorities would have an explicit duty to ensure that the vulnerable clan were protected. In addition to their duties to the individuals comprising the population (which are equally applicable to everyone under their jurisdiction), they have duties towards the African peoples as a unique complex system. The clan, as well as its individual members, should be afforded protection.

Principle (1) above suggests that when a population (as a complex system) is at risk of significant harm (more so than other populations), disproportionate aid should be made available to that population. Just as Rolsten suggests that it would be wrong to intentionally eliminate a wild species of e.g. butterflies in order to improve the monetary value of the few remaining in a collection, so public health has a duty to act to ensure no human populations, such as small vulnerable clans, are abandoned to extinction or subjected to disproportionate harm. This kind of situation is less unusual than one would expect. On the African continent, there are many small peoples arguably deserving of greater attention from a public health perspective than they receive. But the same is true in some areas of the global north, where e.g., Inuit and Metis people live in Canada.

I address principle (2) in greater detail in the next chapter on Decolonising Public Health. Suffice to say for now that many people value their cultural heritage, that this heritage can have pragmatic as well as aesthetic value, and as I will argue in the next chapter, imposing all aspects of the dominant (typically Western) culture on all populations is neither ethical nor health-maximizing. Non-mainstream medicine can undoubtedly be effective, and it's quite plausible that (at least with some conditions) patients could respond better to treatment from healers practicing within a more familiar cultural paradigm.

Principle (3) speaks to progress in respect of attaining the vital goals of the population's members. Whilst protecting cultural heritage is important, improving the health of populations requires the adoption of new, more efficient and effective technologies. Public health policymakers have a duty to ensure these are accessible to the extent possible. Governments must implement fiscal and social policies that help facilitate the rapid development and implementation of new medical, educational, and civil engineering technologies.

Finally, principle (4) concerns the Rawlsian value of liberty, and is related to the "autonomy" principle at the level of the individual. Whilst populations as complex systems do not have agency (since they do not have minds), democratic processes have been developed such that the "will of the people" *en masse* can be respected. Respecting the democratic will of the people is the closest approximation to autonomy I can imagine at the population-scale, and doing so is, I contend, every bit as important as respecting the autonomous choices of individual patients in a clinic. That is not to say that every new public health policy must be subject to a referendum. That would be far too impractical. However, democratic political and legal frameworks should ensure that populations influence the policies and laws imposed on them.

Competing/Conflicting Principles with Population Level Capacities-Based Principlism

Just as the four principles of Beauchamp and Childress's principlism in bioethics sometimes conflict with one another, so the principles of capacities-based principlism at both the level of the individual and at the level of the population may conflict. Principlism in bioethics advocates for Autonomy, Beneficence, Non-Maleficence, and Justice; but if the patient refuses the most effective and harmless treatment, then one cannot simultaneously meet both the autonomy and beneficence/non-maleficence conditions. Similar issues will arise with my proposal in the public health context.

Generally speaking, no patient should be forced into a medical intervention they refuse, unless it is clear that competing principles significantly outweigh the infringement on autonomy. The equivalent at the population level might be a general consensus against a particular public health interventio n, such as a vaccine mandate or a lockdown. This raises an interesting question: should public health policymakers be allowed to enforce general lockdowns or vaccine mandates against the will of the people, on the grounds that it's "for the people's own good".

In the public health context, I'm inclined to think the continued survival and flourishing of populations (maintaining the physical and mental health of its members) can take precedence over the will of the people. This applies to both vaccine mandates and lockdowns. This needs to be done with great care, however. Thorough cost-benefit analyses must be conducted, and experts must have good evidence that restricting the freedoms of the population is necessary. The democratic will of the population might be to never have lockdowns or vaccine mandates, but this could put vulnerable people at risk. The most vulnerable might well be in favour of lockdowns or vaccine mandates, and the population at large not particularly well-versed in the consequences of not doing so. For this reason, the democratic voice I advocate as part of principle (4) should largely pertain to electing those with the ability/knowledge/skills to make well-informed decisions about such matters. In this way, individual decisions that "go against the will of the people" could avoid undermining the overall principle of respecting their collective will.

It is beyond the scope of this chapter to provide precise conditions under which vaccine mandates and lockdowns are, in fact, justified, but as Kass suggests, the potential burdens of the intervention must be weighed up against the benefits. The burdens include (but are not restricted to) the loss of autonomy, the potential side effects on education, the economy and the potential (typically very small) risk to physical and mental health. That said, in my opinion, there are certainly circumstances in which both vaccine mandates and lockdowns can be warranted. A failure to enforce a vaccine mandate, when certain conditions are met, could violate many of the principles proposed by capacities-based principlism on a large scale. When vaccinating protects not only the individual patient but those around them, and when the disease is particularly harmful and transmissible (thus severely affecting the ability of large numbers of people to achieve their vital goals), it might well be worth sacrificing the loss of autonomy.

There can be a similar apparent conflict between the positive (technological and infrastructural) development of populations and preserving cultural heritage. On the face of it, providing modern hospitals undermines Traditional African Medicine (TAM), and building extensive infrastructure (roads, dams, railways, farms) might interfere with the hunter-gatherer practices of certain indigenous groups. Similarly, conflict may arise between preserving cultural heritage and a number of the principles advocated by capacities-based principlism at the individual level. For example, in some African cultures, female genital mutilation (FGM) is common practice (Berg and Denison 2012), and initiation schools for young African males are responsible for hundreds of preventable deaths every year (Mothosola et al. 2019).

I think it important that policymakers ensure that traditional practices are negatively affected to the least extent possible. Some of the Khoi and San peoples continue to live their hunter-gatherer lifestyles in the Kalahari Desert (Barnard 2019), and it would be wrong to prevent them from continuing their chosen lifestyle. Infrastructural improvements must therefore be restricted to those that do not eradicate traditional ways of living.

TAM continues to thrive in the African region, but building hospitals in addition means that individuals have a choice regarding where to receive treatment (often, the answer is both). So long as people are adequately informed about the costs and benefits of both mainstream medicine and TAM, they have the capacity to make autonomous decisions and receive their treatment of choice. I discuss this in more detail in the next chapter, "Decolonizing Public Health".

It is likely no surprise that I am firmly in favour of respecting the capacity of women to make autonomous choices, over promoting the capacity to preserve the cultural heritage of countries where FGM is common practice. In general, the rights of vulnerable individuals within a culture outweigh the duty to preserve the culture. In this instance (on the assumption that most women would not give informed consent to FGM), capacities-based principlism thus advocates for the eradication of FGM.

With respect to initiation practices, whilst capacities-based principlism does not advocate for the abolishment of initiation schools, the lives of those participating must be respected. Those on chronic medication should be able to continue to take their medication during initiation (which is often not allowed), and no young person should be dying of dehydration during initiation (a common cause of death at initiation schools). Appropriate interventions should be taken to prevent these deaths, whilst maintaining the essence of tradition.

It is not possible to produce a consistent hierarchy for the principles of capacities-based principlism. Instead, public health policymakers must consider each decision within its context, and weigh the principles appropriately. When it comes to the principles of capacities-based principlism, I am (again) in broad agreement with what Childress et al. have to say about their "general moral considerations":

> Some argue for a lexical or serial ordering, in which one general moral consideration, Whilst not generally absolute, has priority over another. For instance, one theory might hold that protecting or promoting public health always has priority over privacy, whilst another might hold that individual liberty always has priority over protecting or promoting public health. Neither of these priority rules is plausible, and any priority rule that is plausible will probably involve tight or narrow specifications of the relevant

> general moral considerations to reduce conflicts. From our standpoint, it is better to recognize the need to balance general moral considerations in particular circumstances when conflicts arise. (Childress et al. 2002, p. 172)

In general, these weightings should be determined by public health policymakers in consultation with other stakeholders, with the rights of individuals taking priority. The longer-term consequences of interventions should be prioritized over the short-term implications. For example, the capacity to play can be reasonably outweighed by the long-term goal of saving lives through a short-term lockdown (e.g., following an outbreak of a contagious disease with a high mortality rate, such as Ebola). Similarly, whilst the capacities necessary to preserve cultural heritage are important, any traditions that overtly violate the rights of individuals should be sacrificed, on the assumption that those negatively affected agree to this.

6.10 Conclusion

In this chapter I highlighted the similarities and differences between Venkatapuram's accounts of health and public health ethics and my own, largely in order to both acknowledge his influence on the view developed later in this chapter, and to highlight the benefits of my own approach. I then proposed capacities-based principlism, a framework for public health ethics that outlines the duties of public health decisionmakers to individuals, focusing on the capacities to promote happiness, promote meaning in life, and avoid illness. Whilst most commentators have argued that the policymakers' duties to individuals are exhaustive of those duties, I contend that in addition, policymakers have duties to the population as a complex system/super-organism. I concluded with a further tentative set of principles highlighting what these duties might be.

In the next chapter I develop the idea that policymakers have a duty to preserve (at least some aspects of) cultural heritage. Mainstream medicine is just one of many medical paradigms, and in many countries where mainstream medicine is the only form funded by government, it is not the paradigm indigenous to the region. This has led a number of philosophers to consider whether medicine should be "decolonised", and indeed, what this means (Broadbent 2019b; Harris 2021). Chapter 7 concerns whether public health, too, should be decolonised, and what that might entail.

7

Decolonizing Public Health

7.1 Introduction

In this chapter I look at what it might mean for public health (and the aspects of medicine relevant to public health) to be decolonized, and demonstrate how doing so could significantly improve the health of post-colonial populations. Throughout this book my examples have largely been drawn from Africa, and in particular South Africa. This theme will continue in this chapter, but most of the substantive claims are as applicable to any postcolonial country where indigenous knowledge has been systematically marginalized.

For the last decade or so, "decolonization" (in the metaphorical sense) has become an important aspect of the social and political environment of many postcolonial countries, particularly (although not exclusively) within Africa. In South Africa during the 2015 #feesmustfall protests, the call was for Free Decolonized Education (Griffiths 2019). Whilst it was not made explicitly clear what a decolonized education amounted to, behind the demands were serious and legitimate concerns. Philosophy curricula, for example, mostly comprised nineteenth century Continental/European philosophy and western analytic philosophy, with many

B. Smart, *The Philosophy of Public Health*,
https://doi.org/10.1007/978-3-031-98804-2_7

universities at the time offering little to no African philosophy to African students studying in Africa. A decade later and the situation has changed substantially. Following the pressure of the protests, a wealth of African philosophy from African writers is now being routinely taught nationwide. Similar laudable curricula transformations have occurred in many disciplines/subjects in tertiary education, and the discussion has shifted to whether and how science can be decolonized, how medicine can be decolonized, and so forth.

In Sect. 7.2. I provide a brief introduction to "colonized public health". This section focuses on the role of western approaches to public health in the subjugation of indigenous populations, and the negative effect on their health outcomes. I end the section by considering the impact of epistemic injustice in the medical and public health context in postcolonial societies. In Sect. 7.3. I consider existing ideas in the literature on what it means to decolonize medicine, specifically Alex Broadbent's "Decolonization as Fairness", "Decolonization as Epistemic Equality", and "Critical Decolonization", alongside Chadwin Harris's "Refined Medical Cosmopolitanism", and apply them to the public health context. I highlight some concerns with these views. Finally, in Sect. 7.4. I propose that public health can be decolonized by applying capacities-based principlism (proposed in Chap. 6) through the lens of the marginalized.

7.2 Colonized Public Health: A Brief Introduction

Harris argues that the first step towards decolonizing medicine is to understand the link between medicine and colonialism. What goes for medicine in this respect goes for public health, too. Harris highlights two key issues: "The first aspect is the role medicine played in the spread of empire and the subjugation of colonized people… The second perspective on medicine's culpability in relation to colonialism pertains to the fact that the health outcomes of those at the receiving end of colonialism are worse than those who benefitted from colonialism" (Harris Forthcoming).

With respect to the first aspect, Harris specifies two kinds of examples. The first concerns the abuse of colonized populations in the medical domain. History is rife with examples of targeted oppressed populations being used for inhumane medical experiments. It is well documented, for example, that inhumane medical experimentation took place in the Nazi concentration camps during the second world war, mainly on "gypsies, Jews, Poles and Russians" (Ivy 1947). Unnecessary experimental surgeries were performed on prisoners without their consent, often resulting in death. For example, prisoners were intentionally infected with Typhus in order to test the effectiveness of experimental vaccines, often costing those prisoners their lives (Ivy 1947). The Nazi medical atrocities mostly targeted specific ethnic demographics, in addition to the physically and mentally disabled. But whilst the egregious nature of these crimes is widely acknowledged, perhaps the same cannot be said of similar crimes committed against indigenous populations during, or as a direct result of the colonial era. Harris provides the examples of Sarah Baartman (a Khoi-San woman transported to Europe to showcase anatomical differences between European and African women (Gordon-Chipembere 2011)), the Tuskegee syphilis experiment (in which 600 sons and grandsons of slaves were studied over 40 years without being informed they had a sexually transmitted disease (Thomas and Quinn 2000)), and Dr. James Marion Sims's inhumane gynecological experiments on black female slaves (Khabele et al. 2021). Western medicine "[turned the] colonized environments into a giant laboratory in which to test their hypotheses and speculations" (Harris Forthcoming).

All this, of course, is relevant to public health. But the concerns of population health (in the broad sense discussed in the book) extend beyond medicine and medical research. Wherever colonialism occurred, land was taken by the colonizers, depriving indigenous people of their homes and the means of production. In some cases, political decolonization led to the return of the land. In others, the land (particularly productive farmland) remains predominantly in the hands of the descendants of colonizers (Department of Rural Development and Land Reform 2017).

Historically, many indigenous people from colonized countries were taken as slaves, and their minerals and resources mined and exported to further enrich the west. Colonial rule also resulted in significant negative changes to other areas impacting population health. The apartheid era saw a special curriculum introduced for non-white learners. The "Bantu education", implemented between 1952 and 1992, was "an inferior type of [Christian/European] education that was designed to maintain the subordinate and marginal status of the majority racial group of the country" (Thobejane 2013). Following their education, non-white South Africans were restricted in their employment opportunities, with almost no access to middle-class professions. Non-white populations were also excluded from the democratic process. All this severely affected indigenous population health, and the effects can still be felt to this day.

The second kind of example of the role of medicine in spreading empire and subjugating indigenous populations concerns the appropriation of effective treatments found in non-western medical paradigms (Harding 1997). I discuss shortly how postcolonial societies can rightly be criticized for ignoring the contributions of indigenous medical paradigms, but just as it is wrong to marginalize useful insights from alternative traditions (see Sect. 7.3), it is equally wrong to appropriate effective treatments without compensating those from whom the medical knowledge originates. Examples are plentiful, but include "the rosy periwinkle plant, unique to Madagascar, [which] has been found to contain properties that combat certain cancers. The anti-cancer drugs vincristine and vinblastine have been developed from the periwinkle, resulting in $100 million in annual sales for Eli Lilly and virtually nothing for Madagascar" (Rhot-Arriaza 1996, p. 922).

Beyond Harris's kinds of example lies a third kind: the negative effect of medical colonization on indigenous knowledge—broadly captured through the notion of epistemic injustice. Crudely, epistemic injustices occur where there is unfair treatment of individuals or groups in their capacity as knowers, restricting their capacity to fully participate in knowledge-sharing and decision-making processes. Apartheid, and colonial systems more generally, clearly perpetuate epistemic injustice on a massive scale. I discuss this further in Sect. 7.3.

This section barely scratches the surface of the negative effects of colonization on population health, but the examples above should demonstrate how colonialism systematically violated the principles of capacities-based principlism, as advanced in Chap. 6. At the level of the individual, capacities-based principlism demands that those in power afford everyone the capacity to access employment (with equal opportunities), to access quality education, to access affordable nutritious food, to make autonomous choices, to be politically active, and to be able to express oneself without fear of consequences. Colonialism systematically restricted these capacities for non-white individuals. Similar restrictions on capacities were imposed on non-white populations as complex systems. Contrary to capacities-based principlism, non-white populations were denied the capacity to flourish and develop, their cultural heritage was marginalized, and the collective will of non-white populations was certainly not respected. In short, colonialism sparked public health crises on a massive scale.

Epistemic Injustice in Medicine and Public Health

The now extensive literature in epistemic injustice was arguably initiated by Miranda Fricker's seminal work, *Epistemic Injustice: Power and the Ethics of Knowing* (Fricker 2007). Whilst some ideas contained in this text have been extensively criticized (Beebee 2011), there's little doubt that Fricker brought important and unexplored ethical issues to light.

Fricker divides epistemic injustices into two main categories: testimonial injustice, and hermeneutical injustice. The former concern reducing (credibility deficit) or enhancing (credibility excess) the credibility of a knower based on prejudices based on the knower's identity. Typically, healthy, middle-aged, white, male, cis-gendered heterosexuals are the biggest beneficiaries of credibility excess, and members of marginalized groups are victims of credibility deficit to different extents. Testimonial injustice is widespread in medical practice, since, as Havi Carel and Ian Kidd have convincingly argued:

> …ill people are more vulnerable to testimonial injustice, because they are often regarded as cognitively unreliable, emotionally compromised, or existentially unstable in ways that render their testimonies and interpretations suspect (Carel and Kidd 2014, p. 530)

The latter, hermeneutical injustice, occurs when dominant social groups monopolize interpretation and understanding of experiences, concepts, or events, marginalizing or erasing the perspectives and knowledge of marginalized groups or individuals. Fricker suggests that hermeneutical injustice is a result of conceptual gaps; for example, a patient may lack the medical knowledge to adequately articulate their experience of illness to western medical doctors, and the western doctors might lack the concepts being used by the patient (Carel and Kidd 2014).

Testimonial injustice and hermeneutical injustice have certainly been perpetuated by colonial structures. Eleanor Byrne highlights the structural character of hermeneutical injustice, noting that "a given individual can be a perfectly virtuous listener, yet still be embedded in structures that cause and perpetuate epistemic injustices" (Byrne Forthcoming). This is frequently the case in public health in postcolonial countries, where existing legislation and frameworks tend to marginalize indigenous knowledge. As a result, even where political colonization has ended and members of the indigenous population govern, epistemic injustices continue unabated.

A second "distinct form of epistemic injustice" regularly encountered in postcolonial countries, but not covered by Fricker's original characterization of the problem, is referred to in more recent literature as "willful hermaneutical ignorance" (Pohlhaus 2012):

> Willful hermeneutical ignorance describes instances where marginally situated knowers actively resist epistemic domination through interaction with other resistant knowers, whilst dominantly situated knowers nonetheless continue to misunderstand and misinterpret the world. (Pohlhaus 2012, p. 716)

In cases of willful hermeneutical ignorance, knowers in the marginalized group do not lack the concepts necessary to adequately describe experiences, events, ideas or theories (which Fricker places at the core of hermeneutical injustice); rather, the dominant group refuse to acknowledge these concepts in any meaningful way. Willful hermeneutical ignorance can occur at the level of interacting individuals, but as I will shortly demonstrate, it is perhaps more commonly (certainly in the context of public health) a systemic issue.

In the public health context, willful hermeneutical ignorance often leads to "contributory injustice". As Kristie Dotson explains:

> Contributory injustice is caused by an epistemic agent's situated ignorance, in the form of willful hermeneutical ignorance, in maintaining and utilizing structurally prejudiced hermeneutical resources that result in epistemic harm to the epistemic agency of a knower. Both the structurally prejudiced or biased hermeneutical resources and the agent's situated ignorance are catalysts for contributory injustice. (Dotson 2012, p. 31)

Alex Tate uses the example of a raped woman being interviewed by the police. She is agitated and fails to make eye contact with the policeman—behaviour that any rape-survivor would fully understand. However, the policeman misinterprets this as an indication that the survivor is likely lying. Her contributions are, as a consequence, not taken as seriously as they should be. Tate sets out the conditions for contributory injustice as follows:

> (a) There is a significant gap in the epistemic resources used by a social group *h* with whom *g* regularly interacts,
> (b) This gap prevents members of *h* (but not *g*) from understanding some aspect of *g*'s members' experience,
> (c) This lack of understanding significantly disadvantages or harms members of *g*, and
> (d) This gap occurs and persists due to the epistemic marginalisation of *g*. (Tate 2019, p. 98)

Contributory injustice, as characterized by Tate, was found to be commonplace in psychiatry, where patients regularly feel as though the rigid frameworks within which (western) mental healthcare practitioners operate exclude the unique experiences of the patient (Tate 2019, p. 99). Diagnosis in this context requires fairly well-defined boxes to be ticked, but often the experiences of patients don't quite fit the boxes. Given that indigenous populations in postcolonial societies such as South Africa have an entirely different understanding of the mechanisms of disease (for example, "amafufunyana", a condition symptomatically identical to schizophrenia, is understood in spiritual terms—caused either by witchcraft, or by the ancestors "calling" the patient to become a traditional healer (Ngubane and DeGama 2024)), contributory injustice in Tate's sense is likely to be particularly prevalent in postcolonial societies, where "gaps" (borrowing from Tate), or rather "differences" in epistemic resources are more extreme.

On the face of it, neither Dotson nor Tate's characterization of contributory injustice captures all "contributory" epistemic harms endured by postcolonial populations. Notably, in the public health context, the failure to adopt indigenous knowledge systems into public policy. In postcolonial countries, those in power are often not ignorant of the marginalized epistemologies—they are members of the marginalized communities. Thus, the (contributory) epistemic harms endured by the indigenous populations do not come about through a failure of those in positions of power to understand the excluded indigenous epistemic resources, but through a failure to incorporate these resources into publicly funded programmes.[1] Abraham Tobi refers to this phenomenon as "intra-group epistemic injustice" (Tobi 2023). I speak to this more in Sect. 7.4.

Whilst it is beyond the scope of this chapter to provide a comprehensive analysis of epistemic injustice in postcolonial countries, it should be clear that colonialism, and the resultant power dynamics in postcolonial countries, has given rise to widespread epistemic injustice in a variety of forms. Indeed, whilst in the next section I consider a number of ways (some unrelated to epistemic issues) in which public health can be

[1] I acknowledge that one might argue that "contributory injustice" is *defined* (by Dotson) in part as being caused by willful hermeneutical ignorance, and thus all cases of contributory injustice are (*de dicto*) necessarily caused by willful hermeneutical ignorance—but since the form of epistemic injustice I describe involves the contribution (or lack thereof) of epistemic resources, and the effect is the same (the exclusion of indigenous knowledge), contributory injustice seems like an appropriate category. Further, as Veli Mitova noted in private correspondence, one might "reject the claim that situated ignorance is involved. It is not ignorance of the traditional medicine… but of its rightful epistemic authority. Here we can talk about internalized colonial thinking." Whilst I agree with Prof Mitova that this may sometimes be the case, I still contend that there have been those in positions of power in South Africa ignorant neither of traditional African medicine, nor of its proper epistemic authority.

decolonized, I take addressing epistemic injustice to be at the core of decolonization.

7.3 What Does It Mean to Decolonize Public Health?

Decolonization in contemporary discourse is a metaphorical notion. In the literal sense, colonization largely ended across Africa and Asia at various points during the twentieth century. But clearly, the footprints of colonialism remain, in some cases (as in South Africa) in the form of racial demographics, but more importantly with respect to the effects of colonialism on culture, language, economics, politics, industry, education, legal systems, religion, healthcare, and wealth and land distribution, and so on. When I speak of decolonization in this chapter, I refer to addressing the persisting negative effects of colonialism on population health. In this section, I explore existing conceptions of decolonization in the context of medicine (extrapolating to public health), considering the extent to which they are consistent with capacities-based principlism.

Let us divide the issues pertinent to decolonization into two primary categories. The first I refer to as the *Epistemic Category*, and the second the *Inequality Category*.

The Epistemic Category

George Khufsh argues that "epistemologies" can be divided into three categories: descriptive epistemology, normative epistemology, and meta-epistemology. Work in descriptive epistemology concerns the way in which people obtain and use knowledge—it describes the decision-making processes and reasoning strategies of epistemic agents. Normative epistemology concerns how epistemic agents *should* obtain and use knowledge; that is, what epistemic agents consider good justification for their beliefs, and when these beliefs can justifiably be translated into e.g. treatment plans. Meta-epistemology involves investigation into descriptive and normative epistemology (Khushf 2013, pp. 463–464).

Let us take epistemic colonization to occur when indigenous knowledge systems such as TAM are marginalized and replaced or dominated by their colonial counterparts. This occurs through a variety of processes. Sometimes intentionally (e.g. during apartheid South Africa), and sometimes through the less malicious, but equally problematic, implicit biases (crudely, the unconscious, unintentional, and often subtle attitudes or stereotypes that affect our judgements, decisions, and interactions with others, at the expense of marginalized groups) of those in positions of power. Epistemic colonization thus comes about, at least in part, through testimonial injustice and contributory injustice, as discussed above. Epistemic decolonization would be the process of reversing epistemic colonization.

Epistemic Decolonization and Traditional African Medicine

The diversity in medical paradigms highlights how extensively medical epistemologies can differ. In diagnosing mental health conditions, for example, those working in mainstream medicine will refer to the diagnostic criteria contained in the DSM-5. They will look for reasonably well-specified physical, psychological, and behavioural symptoms identified through extensive studies (descriptive epistemology), and often try to work within the preferred evidence based medicine (EBM) framework when it comes to treatment plans (normative epistemology). Sangomas working in Traditional African Medicine (TAM) will, instead, use the process of divination. In their consultation with the patient, they will "throw the bones", read meaning into the way they land, and communicate with the ancestors to determine the cause of their patient's ill health and the appropriate treatment (Audet et al. 2021). Clearly, there is much intercultural disagreement between mainstream and African medicine with respect to both the reasoning processes (descriptive epistemology), and how those practitioners think one *should* come to obtain "medical knowledge".

Despite the continued popularity of TAM in South Africa, with an estimated 70–80% of the population making use of that medical paradigm (Peltzer 2009), TAM receives no government funding. Government-funded clinics and hospitals exclusively practice mainstream western medicine. Many would no doubt argue that this is rational. "After all…" (they might say) "…mainstream medicine works, and other forms of medicine are quackery. Why should the taxpayer fund ineffective medicine?"

Were it true that mainstream medicine is always highly effective, that TAM and other non-western medical paradigms are entirely ineffective, and that this fully explains the adoption of mainstream medicine and exclusion of TAM, then there might be little to complain about. However, none of these things are true. Mainstream medicine is not always highly effective, there's good reason to think other medical paradigms can help sick patients (at least for some conditions), and the discrepancy in effectiveness (regardless of what that is) does not fully explain TAM's exclusion. The epistemic colonization of medicine is therefore, at least on the face of it, unjust.

What goes for medicine in this context, goes for much of public health policy. Public health policy, both on the broad and narrow understandings of public health advanced in this book (those that include e.g. education, and those pertaining exclusively to physical health), is determined by those in positions of power, and the political and social structures (including legislation/constitutions etc.) under which they operate. Following colonization and later Apartheid in South Africa, the power structures are such that TAM and many other indigenous knowledge systems pertaining to population health in the broader sense have been marginalized.

Systemic epistemic colonization and the corresponding contributory injustices, has significant consequences. It results in a loss of cultural diversity, the erosion of traditional knowledge, the marginalization of indigenous voices, and the reinforcement of dominant power structures at the expense of the marginalized. All these consequences run counter to the ethical principles of capacities-based principlism, both at the individual and population levels presented in Chap. 6.

The Inequality Category

In addition to epistemic colonization, colonialism has shaped the structure of economies and distribution of wealth. In some countries, the negative economic effects of colonialism on indigenous populations are very obvious. According to the World Bank, South Africa is the most unequal country in the world (The World Bank 2022), with the majority of white South Africans sitting comfortably in the middle class, and the majority of black/non-white South Africans living in poverty, or at least significantly less comfortably than the middle class. Further, one of the big political debates since the end of apartheid concerns land distribution. Whilst it is beyond the scope of this chapter to engage in this debate, it is worth noting that according to the South African government's 2017 land audit report, 72% of farmland and agricultural holdings are owned by white farmers (Department of Rural Development and Land Reform 2017), when at the time of writing only 7.3% of South Africa's population is white (StatsSA 2022).

Wealth and income inequality have an enormous impact on the health of populations. In addition to substantive income discrepancies between the top 10% (or so) of earners and the rest, South Africa has the highest unemployment rate in the world, with the vast majority of the unemployed being people of colour. As I've argued in previous chapters, unemployment seriously impacts the health of populations. In addition to the obvious effects of poverty on nutrition and housing, it deprives people of a source of meaning.

South Africa undeniably has a two-tier healthcare system, with the 16% of the population using private medical facilities receiving world class medical care, and the rest (using free government healthcare services) receiving an extremely poor service (at least with respect to mainstream medicine). The effects of income and wealth inequality in South Africa thus extend to health inequalities. Currently, around the same amount of money is spent on the 16% with medical aid, as is spent on the 84% using government facilities, and as mentioned, 100% of government funding goes towards western mainstream medicine. Furthermore, reports of corruption and wastage in the public health sector are not uncommon, leading to even less money-per-capita being used for actual services/treatment. Progress has been made since the days of apartheid, but an unacceptable degree of racial inequality remains.

This situation is not unique to South Africa. Indeed, sometimes discrepancies in treatment between racial categories cannot be put down to financial considerations. Implicit bias demonstrably plays a significant role in clinical decision making. In the United States, a study showed a notable anti-black bias with respect thrombolysis decisions in patients with acute coronary syndromes (see Smart 2017, p. 5). A study by Schulman *et al* further showed that black women were significantly less likely to receive cardiac catheterization than white women with the same symptoms (Schulman et al. 1999). In these cases, it is not access to adequate primary care that explains the inequality, but anti-black implicit bias, and perhaps hermaneutical injustice, too.

These kinds of inequalities violate the Rawlsian principles grounding capacities-based principlism, and in South Africa, are at least in part a result of colonialism and apartheid. Reducing these inequalities might well be considered part of the decolonial project. With that in mind, let us consider what decolonization entails.

Decolonization as Fairness

Alex Broadbent presents three possible interpretations of what it might mean to decolonize medicine, the first of which is "Decolonization as Fairness" (Broadbent 2019a, p. 245). This approach directly addresses the Inequality Category highlighted above, suggesting that to decolonize is to "redouble efforts to universalize access… [More] needs to be invested in public hospitals, or else realistically affordable insurance schemes need to be developed, or some other public initiative to solve this problem needs to be undertaken" (Broadbent 2019b, p. 247). By "universalizing access", Broadbent is referring to access to mainstream medicine. This would not address the implicit bias issues noted above—that would require additional measures such as strict adherence to evidence based practice, and perhaps awareness programmes for clinicians. Nor would it address the issue of epistemic colonization, but it should at least improve health outcomes for marginalized groups.

Expanded to the public health context, Decolonization as Fairness would entail, in addition to access to curative and preventative medical care, the universal provision of clean water, safe public transportation, adequate sanitation including (in the South African context) the elimination of e.g. pit toilets in government schools, and on the broader definition of population health adopted in this book, the provision of quality education for all learners, and access to employment opportunities. All laudable goals in line with capacities-based principlism.

The trouble with Decolonization as Fairness, and the reason Broadbent himself rejects it, is that whilst it helps deals with the inequality effect of colonialism, it fails to address the Epistemic Category. Ensuring everyone in a post-colonial country has access to quality healthcare, sanitation, clean water, education, and jobs, does nothing (in itself) to promote the adoption of marginalized indigenous knowledge systems. "The people who do the providing also decide what to provide. We may be equalizing one aspect – equality of access—but the underlying power relations remain along the lines as they were, and may be amplified" (Broadbent 2019a, p. 247). In short, whilst promoting "fairness" in access to quality medical care, and ensuring the positive effects of public health interventions are ubiquitous, is certainly something policymakers should strive for, this alone would be insufficient to complete the decolonial project in public health.

Decolonization as Epistemic Equality

Broadbent labels his second approach to decolonizing medicine: Decolonization as Epistemic Equality. "On this view, the knowledge claims of different medical traditions must be taken equally seriously" (Broadbent 2019b, p. 251). Epistemic equality requires policymakers to pay equal attention to both the descriptive and normative epistemologies of the different cultures, essentially uncritically accepting the truth of all claims to medical knowledge (or at least acting as if they are true). Tricky, when they frequently contradict one another.

In short, were Broadbent's epistemic equality embraced, clinical guidelines in the South African context would have to incorporate both the western approaches to diagnosis, and traditional divination strategies. They would have to regard the spiritual ways of the Sangoma, and randomized controlled trials and observational studies, as equally valid strategies for obtaining medical knowledge. The same goes for treatment strategies.

Arguably, Broadbent's Epistemic Equality wouldn't be true decolonization, in the sense that the imposed western epistemologies would still be given equal weighting. A more comprehensive approach (which could not be labelled "Decolonization as Epistemic Equality") might be to replace western mainstream medicine with TAM altogether—complete "Africanization".

Much like Decolonization as Fairness, Decolonization as Epistemic Equality can be roughly translated into the public health context by exporting this attitude towards differing epistemologies to any issue lying in the domain of public health. Traditional African approaches to education (both in terms of pedagogy and curricula), governance, agriculture, sanitation, and so forth would, under this approach, be given equal consideration as the dominant western approaches.

Broadbent rightly notes that this approach gives rise to "wholesale relativism" about medicine and medical knowledge, a position he rejects on the grounds of the harm such an approach can cause, both to humans and other animals. For example, ground rhino horn is a traditional Chinese remedy, dating back centuries, for fever, hangovers, poisoning, and more recently for erectile dysfunction. It's possible (given the psychological underpinnings of a large proportion of those suffering from erectile dysfunction) that using ground rhino horn has the desired effect from time to time. But rhino horn is primarily composed of Keratin (the same protein found in human fingernails), Calcium phosphate, Calcium carbonate, and Magnesium phosphate. No constituent of rhino horn could have any (non-placebo) effect that could help with erectile dysfunction. Nonetheless, African rhino horn sells for vast sums of money, and the resultant rhino poaching in Africa has left the poor rhinoceros on the brink of extinction.

The pending (likely) extinction of rhinos through misguided medical beliefs in Traditional Chinese Medicine is shocking enough. But whilst I do not wish to dwell on the negative aspects of TAM, it's worth noting that certain beliefs propagated by some traditional healers have caused enormous suffering. For example, Suzanne Leclerc-Madlala has written on how (some) traditional healers in South Africa instructed their HIV-infected patients to have sexual intercourse with a virgin in order to prevent AIDS. A nationwide survey of 9000 young South Africans in 2002 showed that 13% of participants believed this to be an effective intervention. This has been identified as a possible factor in the rape of thousands of babies and children in South Africa (Leclerc-Madlala 2002). Needless-to-say, raping virgins has no effect on the progression of the disease, except insofar as many of the victims become infected, too.

It would be inappropriate for me to use these examples without highlighting (again) the damage caused by Mainstream Medicine. As discussed in Chap. 3, thousands of children were born with underdeveloped limbs after their mothers took Thalidomide to help with morning sickness (Kim and Scialli 2011). And this, of course, is not the only example. Western mainstream medicine is not immune from causing harm, even with the shift towards evidence-based medicine in the 1990s.

Unsurprisingly, Broadbent concludes that Epistemic Equality is not the right path to a decolonized medicine, and of course I agree. It solves some of the epistemic colonization problems, but the cost is far too high.

Critical Decolonization

Broadbent's answer to decolonizing medicine is "Critical Decolonization".

> …critical decolonization means accepting risk of error. It means considering whether the canon might be wrong… It also means asking whether ancestors really cause disease, or care about slaughtered goats. Indigenous knowledge systems might contain truths that Western science has not accessed. This is uncomfortable for Western science. But indigenous knowledge systems might also be wrong, either partially and understandably, or totally and extravagantly… The goal of critical decolonization is to get to the truth, and nobody gets a free pass. (Broadbent 2019a, p. 259)

For Broadbent, to endorse Critical Decolonization is to adopt what he calls "Medical Cosmopolitanism". This is reducible to four distinct "stances": a metaphysical stance, an epistemic stance, a moral stance, and a commitment to the "primacy of practice" (Broadbent 2019b, pp. 181–207). Briefly, the metaphysical stance commits one to realism; that is, medical facts are universally applicable. That's not to say, of course, that if a drug works for one person it works for all; rather, that if certain exposures cause disease, then they do so mind-independently. If supernatural beings cause disease, they do so mind-independently. The metaphysical stance is essentially the rejection of medical relativism.

The epistemic stance is a commitment to epistemic humility. One should accept that one's views may be false (in a broadly Popperian, falsificationist sense), be open to further testing of one's beliefs, and changing them when the evidence suggests one should. Broadbent notes that this is equally applicable to evidential standards. As I will argue shortly, I think this issue lies at the heart of the problem with Critical Decolonization.

The moral stance states that all individuals should be taken to have equal moral worth. Perhaps this seems trivial in the modern era in the West, but certainly less trivial in postcolonial countries where, as we have seen, the moral stance has frequently (and recently) been violated.

Finally, primacy of practice advocates that medical practitioners should focus on implementing effective interventions, rather than on the truth of explanations for why patients are diseased and why the interventions work. For example, acupuncture from the Chinese tradition involves inserting thin needles into specific points of the body. It is recognized as (at least possibly) an effective treatment for various forms of pain (Lam and Galvin 2013), but the underlying theory involves appeal to "meridian lines", also known as "qi" or "energy pathways", through which life energy flows (Ho 2006). When qi becomes "blocked or imbalanced", disease follows. Acupuncture, according to traditional Chinese belief systems, restores balance by clearing blockages, excesses, or deficiencies in qi. Western medicine does not recognize the existence of qi; but, according to Broadbent, this should not matter. The primacy of practice advocates that should acupuncture work as pain relief, it should be used—irrespective of the theory that grounds it.

Critical decolonization, through medical cosmopolitanism, has its benefits. On the face of it, it resolves the epistemic inequality issue, since it demands both critical analysis of the dominant paradigm (epistemic humility), and serious consideration of the causal and treatment claims of alternative medical (or in the context of this book, broader public health) paradigms. The moral stance goes some way to addressing the issue of inequality, too.

I foresee problems with critical decolonization, however. "Western medicine" and "Western public health", as paradigms, are not simply reducible to the problems they recognize, the causes of the problems they recognize, and the interventions they recognize. They include methodological considerations: standards of evidence, strategies for obtaining evidence of effectiveness, and the evidence deemed necessary for informed policy decision-making, such as those offered by evidence-based medicine and evidence-based public health. Broadbent's critical decolonization asks that we "get to the truth", but this requires a methodology for getting to the truth. Traditional African Medicine deems divination a truth-conducive methodology. Western medicine does not.

The western mindset will no doubt suggest that the effectiveness of non-western interventions can be tested through clinical trials (or similar strategies in other fields) just as easily as western interventions. Whilst some have argued that it is unethical to continue to use e.g. Traditional African Medicine without "concerted efforts to improve efficacy and safety" through scientific research (Nyika 2009, p. S32), others will claim this approach fails to account for the inherently spiritualist nature of many alternative paradigms. Sangomas might reasonably argue that "being put to the test" in this way itself undermines the effectiveness of the intervention.

Whilst Broadbent recognizes this issue when he asserts that "unlike (most) EBM-ers, our conception of evidence must be likewise humble; it is no use being willing to test anything, but adamantine in one's refusal to consider whether one's evidential standards are correct or appropriate" (Broadbent 2019a, p. 204), it seems extraordinarily unlikely that those embedded in the western tradition will accept the evidential standards of TAM. As Harris notes, "what do we say to the traditional healer who insists that the ancestor-wrath explanation for TB is supported by evidence, namely the fact that this was the diagnosis conveyed to him in a dream or in a trance state?" (Harris Forthcoming). I am reminded of Broadbent's own response to decolonization as Epistemic Equality, where he quotes Kwame Appiah:

> One may be reminded of an old story from the colonial days of India. A British officer who was trying to stop a suttee was told by an Indian man. "It's our custom to burn a widow on her husband's funeral pyre." To which the officer replied, "And it's our custom to execute murders." (Appiah 2007, p. 24)

In short, trying to reach a consensus on "the truth" from different traditions will prove exceptionally difficult, since the evidential standards of those involved are ultimately irreconcilable.

Harris's Refined Cosmopolitanism

Harris argues that Broadbent's metaphysical and epistemic stances are ultimately incompatible. To rectify the impasse, he proposes that the core of the epistemic stance be changed from epistemic humility, to "striving for objectivity" (Harris Forthcoming). Whilst there are objective medical facts (concerning e.g., which interventions are effective), these facts, or rather, beliefs in these facts, can be arrived at from a plurality of epistemic perspectives.

Drawing from Appiah, Harris uses the "oft-told anecdote about a medical missionary in a remote place" (Appiah 2007), where mothers were giving their infants dirty water to drink and consequently their infants were getting diarrhea. The missionary explained how boiling water kills the microbes causing the diarrhea, but this had no effect on the behaviour of the mothers. However, when the missionary changed the story to accommodate the indigenous population's epistemic framework, by telling the mothers the illness was caused by evil spirits (and that when the water was boiled you could see the spirits bubbling out), the mothers acted fast. They started to boil the water, and the prevalence of diarrhea among the infants dropped significantly.

For Harris, this highlights the distinction between objective medical facts (that boiling water helps prevents disease), and the different ways in which these facts can be interpreted. Arguably, both medicine and public health are results-orientated disciplines; that is to say, what matters is whether the interventions are effective, that there is broad agreement on this, and that the uptake among the population (where relevant) is good. Whether everyone agrees on the mechanisms underlying the interventions is of considerably less importance.

Unsurprisingly, Harris encourages us to consider the notion of objectivity itself. Scientific "knowledge", as it's normally understood, is embedded in the culture of western science. Its goals, assumptions, methodologies, and ultimately its conclusions are value-laden; that is, they are laden with the values of the west. For (strong) objectivity,

> we must become adept at turning the producers of scientific knowledge into the object of scientific knowledge... and make it a priority of medicine to start scientific enquiry from the perspective of marginalized lives, in other words from the perspective of the lives that were "devalued and neglected" during the course of colonialism. (Harris Forthcoming)

All this, of course, extends to the context of public health. I discussed in previous chapters how foreseeably problematic the COVID-19 lockdown in South Africa was. Families living hand-to-mouth, with breadwinners working in the informal sector, were ordered not to leave their residences to work. Obeying that order would mean no food, so of course the order was largely ignored. This public health intervention resulted in making criminals of the poor alongside significant police brutality, with very few, if any, public health benefits. This intervention was not considered from the perspective of marginalized lives (Broadbent et al. 2020; Harris Forthcoming).

Given the Rawlsian principles this book largely assumes, and the two varieties of capacities-based principlism I derive from these underlying Rawlsian tenets, I am drawn to Harris's idea. It promotes the capacities of both individuals and populations, whilst respecting indigenous knowledge systems and cultural values. But whilst Harris is more explicit in his recommendation that multiple epistemic perspectives driving towards the same effective interventions could be endorsed than Broadbent, I suspect Broadbent might respond that this is perfectly compatible with his epistemic stance. Perhaps Harris would not disagree (after all, he calls the view "refined cosmopolitanism"). The problem, it seems to me, is that the primary issue with Broadbent's epistemic stance remains unresolved. The primary problems concern the irreconcilable differences in evidential standards.

In the missionary example, above, the lead is taken from western medicine. The "boiling the water" intervention derives from the western understanding of the germ theory of disease, and our mechanistic knowledge that boiling water kills the harmful microorganisms causing illness. Charitably put, the missionary translates this medical knowledge into the epistemic perspective of the indigenous population. Less charitably, the missionary lies in order to coerce the population into adopting their intervention, effective and medically beneficial as it was.

The missionary's approach, extrapolated (perhaps to the extreme) in a public health context, entails adopting western public health interventions, "translating" the mechanisms of the intervention into concepts more easily acceptable to indigenous populations, and encouraging those populations to adopt those interventions. If the evidential standards of alternative paradigms (such as divination) are rejected, medical cosmopolitanism (refined or otherwise), and its public health counterpart, would likely continue to be (almost) exclusively dominated by western interventions; that is, the interventions deemed fit by the dominant social structures.

I endorse the general rejection of medical relativism. I believe that, despite significant variation between individuals (and thus two distinct individuals will often react differently to the same intervention), there are medical facts. HIV causes AIDS (and antiretroviral therapy is an effective intervention); smoking tobacco causes lung cancer, and so forth. Nonetheless, I also believe that alternative medicine has an enormous amount to offer that is unjustly marginalized by governments and big pharmaceutical companies, as are many insights from indigenous knowledge systems relevant to public health more broadly—all at the expense of human populations. In the next section, I present my approach to decolonizing public health, which, it will come as no surprise, draws on

Rawlsian principles and focuses on promoting the capacities of marginalized populations.

7.4 Capacities-Based Decolonization

In Chap. 6, I argued that public health policymakers and workers have a duty to promote the following capacities for individuals:

1. The capacity to access safe, affordable housing;
2. The capacity to access electricity;
3. The capacity to access clean, running water and sanitation;
4. The capacity to access employment (when necessary, with equal opportunities, and adequate pay);
5. The capacity to access affordable, nutritious food;
6. The capacity to access quality education;
7. The capacity to access quality preventative and curative medical interventions;
8. The capacity to freely express oneself without fear of consequences (excluding hate speech);
9. The capacity to make autonomous choices (that do not infringe on the rights of others);
10. The capacity to be politically active (e.g. to protest, to vote, to be elected);
11. The capacity to move freely, and safely, at least within one's own country;
12. The capacity to live (maximally) free of crime and/or the fear of crime;
13. The capacity to live (maximally) free from discrimination (racial/sexual/gender, etc.);
14. The capacity to form loving relationships;
15. The capacity to play;
16. The capacity to appreciate/enjoy aesthetic value (participate in the arts, be a spectator of the arts/sports, access natural beauty, etc.)

And the following capacities at the population level:

1. Promote the capacities necessary for the continued survival and flourishing of populations as complex systems.
2. Promote the capacities necessary for the preservation of the cultural heritage of populations as complex systems (should this be 'the collective will of the people').
3. Promote the capacities necessary for the positive development (technological, infrastructural, etc.) of populations as complex systems.
4. Promote the capacities necessary for the collective will (in the democratic sense) of populations as complex systems to be respected (where this does not violate the rights of individuals).

I further argued that promoting these capacities was the way to realize the Rawlsian principles of equality, freedom, and solidarity through: (1) ensuring, to the extent possible, that individuals have the capacity to maximally prevent and/or cure physical and mental disorders; and (2) ensuring, to the extent possible, that individuals have the capacity to live maximally meaningful, happy, pain-free lives. I contend that decolonizing public health means addressing both inequality and epistemic colonization by promoting these capacities "from the perspective of the lives that were "devalued and neglected" during the course of colonialism" (Harris Forthcoming). Let us now apply this approach to the two core themes of decolonization: The Inequality Category, and The Epistemic Category.

7.5 Capacities-Based Decolonization and Inequality

Capacities-based principlism, both at the individual and population level, is designed to promote the Rawlsian values of liberty, equality, and solidarity, in part through the equitable distribution of social goods. The capacities I outline above should be considered social goods, and of course striving towards the equal distribution of these capacities would help address the issue of inequality. In postcolonial countries, decolonization with respect to inequality would involve directly addressing any inequalities arising from colonialism, and in truth, this likely refers to most inequalities experienced in postcolonial countries. As discussed in Chap. 6, capacities-based principlism advocates these duties (that is, advancing the capacities of the disadvantaged) irrespective of the causal base; that is, whilst the inequalities are a side-effect of colonialism, and thus addressing them forms a part of the decolonial project, public health (government, public health workers, and arguably corporations engaging in "corporate social responsibility") would have a duty to address these inequalities regardless of what caused them. As Harris notes, though, the decolonial project demands that this should be done through the lens of the disadvantaged.

In this book, I have largely focused on government interventions, but governments are not the only institutions capable of contributing to population health. Large corporations with a moral (and sometimes legal) obligation to engage in corporate social responsibility (CSR) programmes also have a role to play. For example, since 2016, Microsoft has donated USD25,000,000 to over 2300 non-profits in South Africa to help bridge the digital divide (MicrosoftNewsCentre 2018). But it's no use addressing the digital divide by providing computers to schools that lack the infrastructure (e.g., access to electricity) necessary to use them. Those computers will end up in landfill (I'm not suggesting Microsoft or any of the non-profits they funded did this, but anecdotally, precisely this mistake has been made in the past through similar programmes).

Those organizing CSR programmes must consult with all stakeholders—including those who will benefit from the programmes—to ensure that the needs of the indigenous community are met in a way that's consistent with their values. Communities "benefitting" from CSR frequently don't feel this is this case. A member of the mining community at Marikana, for example, had this to say about the recreational facility the mining company built at a nearby town as part of their CSR programme:

> The location of the recreational facility is not appropriate because our community does not have a football or other sporting facilities where our young people can gather to socialize outside of their school premises. As a result of boredom, young people [both male and female] use 'myaope' [drug] and

> congregate at local taverns during weekends and holidays. They overlooked us in locating the facility because we cannot pay for its use, unlike the residents of the town where the facility is located (Samuel and Mqomboti 2017, pp. 62–63).

Building a recreational facility is a wonderful example of how corporations can promote the capacities of the population. It provides the capacity to improve physiological health, the capacity to play, and sports can provide a source of meaning in life. However, clearly the residents near the mine felt the facility is too far away (and perhaps too expensive) to address their needs. The facility allows the company to advertise their wonderful CSR programme, but does not improve the health (broadly construed) of their employees' families.

A key component of successful CSR programmes, then, is a thorough consultative process with the communities involved. The needs and desires and cultural context of the community must be assessed, and the programmes must directly address those needs and desires. This consultative principle is equally applicable to the interventions of government and non-profit organizations. For example, the problems encountered by the World Bank's child nutrition project in Bangladesh, where the successful interventions implemented in Tamil Nadu (of educating mothers in child nutrition and providing food supplements) were replicated, but failed (Cartwright 2013), could have been avoided had the mothers been interviewed more thoroughly prior to implementation.

In short, applying capacities-based principlism at the individual and population level will directly address (and go some way to resolving) the Inequality Category of decolonization—but decolonial interventions must involve the participation of the marginalized through a productive consultative process.

7.6 Capacities-Based Principlism and the Epistemic Category

Perhaps the capacity most relevant to avoiding epistemic harms in capacities-based principlism at the individual level, is the capacity to live (maximally) free from discrimination. Discrimination, for the purposes of this project, goes beyond explicit racism, sexism, racism, ageism, and so on, and extends into the realm of implicit biases and epistemic injustices (which may be a consequence of explicit prejudices, or implicit biases). Ensuring the capacity to live free from discrimination thus entails public health should help address all the above issues.

Other capacities highlighted at the individual level are less obviously linked to epistemic decolonization, but nonetheless are. The capacity to access quality education, for example, is inherently linked to epistemic decolonization. In a postcolonial country, a "quality" education must be a decolonized education. It is beyond the scope of this chapter to provide a thorough explanation of what a decolonized education amounts to, and (as a white immigrant from the west) I am perhaps not the person best fitted to providing such an account. However, it is fairly obvious that restricting one's curricula to authors and content from the west is not appropriate in the South African context; educators must be mindful of the fact that students typically do not have English as a first language, and should accommodate this fact in their pedagogical strategies; educators should also be cognizant of testimonial injustice and their implicit biases.[2]

Population-level capacities-based principlism (see Chap. 6.) is in its entirety is relevant to epistemic decolonization. Populations cannot flourish if their members are enduring persistent epistemic harms. An integral part of preserving the cultural heritage of populations involves preserving and promoting indigenous knowledge systems. Positive development of these communities should include the development and implementation of effective indigenous knowledge, and the collective will of indigenous populations will typically involve requiring public health policymakers

[2] For further ideas pertaining to decolonizing education, certainly in the African context, I recommend Norah Barongo-Muweke's book: *Decolonizing Education: Towards Reconstructing a Theory of Citizenship Education for Postcolonial Africa* (2016).

and stakeholders to be respectful and cognizant of indigenous belief systems, ways of life, and their context-specific needs. Again, achieving the four principles of population-level capacities-based principlism requires significant engagement of public health policymakers and stakeholders (such as companies with CSR programmes) with communities, to understand their needs.

Let us now consider potential solutions to the epistemic injustices outlined earlier in this chapter. I consider three distinct problems in turn. The first is testimonial injustice, where knowers (perhaps patients, or those in need in need of public health interventions) are victims of credibility deficit; the second is hermeneutical injustice in Fricker's sense, where knowers lack the theoretical concepts necessary to explain their experiences and needs to those in positions of power (e.g. doctors and public health officials); the third is willful hermeneutical ignorance and relatedly contributory injustice, where indigenous knowledge systems are marginalized despite their potential uses. The first two I address here through Havi Carel and Ian Kidd's "toolkit" for epistemic injustice in medicine.

Carel and Kidd propose a toolkit for addressing epistemic injustice in the medical context: a phenomenological approach. This comprises three stages: "bracketing the natural attitude towards illness", which "suspends the belief in the reality of the disease entity"; "thematizing illness [which] refers to the act of attending to a phenomenon in a way that makes particular aspects of it explicit [e.g., the cognitive, emotive, moral, or aesthetic aspects of a phenomenon"; and, "reviewing the ill person's being in the world… [which] take[s] the new understanding of illness emerging from [the first] two steps, and examine[s] how it changes one's being in the world." (Carel and Kidd 2014, p. 538)

> This toolkit uses being in the world to capture the pervasive effects illness may have on one's sense of place, on one's interactions with the environment and with other people, on meanings and norms, and on the nexus of entities, habits, knowledge, and other people that makes up one's world. [It] enables participants to move away from a narrow understanding of illness as a biological process, towards a thick account of illness as a new way of being in the world. (Carel and Kidd 2014, p. 538)

Carel and Kidd's solution (which they themselves highlight as just one possible measure) is, perhaps to put it overly simply, to prioritise the patient's lived experience over the biological reality of disease. To some extent, a move away from EBM (although, as outlined in Chap. 3, EBM does also highlight the importance of patient-values), and towards a specific iteration of patient-centered care.

It's worth noting the following challenge: in order for this to work, doctors must be able to comprehend the patient's descriptions of the cognitive, emotive, moral and aesthetic experiences of illness. In postcolonial contexts, western-trained physicians with no experience of e.g., indigenous African culture, may not be best placed to understand these descriptions. Whilst patients (often) lack the epistemic resources to describe their illness in "scientific" terms, physicians trained in mainstream medicine (often) lack the epistemic resources to understand traditional African concepts pertaining to the experience of illness. Bearing in mind the importance of the decolonial project in promoting capacities-based principlism, the onus, it seems to me, falls on the medical professional. Medical practitioners have a (moral) duty to learn indigenous illness-related concepts currently alien to them, just as we all had a duty to grasp concept of "sexual harassment" when that hermeneutical gap was finally filled (Fricker 2007).

Overall, I largely endorse Carel and Kidd's suggestions (which ultimately tie in well with Harris's). If doctors have a better grasp of the patient's experience, and learn how to interpret the concepts they employ, then they are better placed to determine whether patients are making genuinely autonomous choices—one of the principles of capacities-based principlism—when agreeing to medical interventions. Guidelines ensuring that the patient-perspective is placed front and centre, alongside grasping the concepts they employ, should mitigate against both testimonial injustice and hermeneutical injustice. Their strategy does not marginalize indigenous cultures/ways of understanding illness, but rather embraces them.

This phenomenological approach to medical practice can be extended to other areas concerning public health. Decolonizing education and mitigating against epistemic injustice in that sphere should involve the participation of students and their families; educators need to understand the "cognitive, emotive, moral, or aesthetic aspects" of their educational experience (and the causes thereof) in order to make appropriate changes to the curricula and/or pedagogical methods. The same applies for more general public health concerns: environmental pollution (noise pollution, air pollution, waste, etc.) experienced by local communities, access (or lack thereof) to recreational facilities, access to education—indeed, anything pertaining to the capacities outlined in capacities-based principlism. Stakeholders in public health decisions must engage in a thorough consultative process, where the phenomenological experiences of the marginalized are emphasized and understood using the epistemic resources of the marginalized. Only then can appropriate interventions be pursued.

Finally, I come to the contributory injustice issue; that through willful hermeneutical ignorance, the epistemic resources of the marginalized are sidelined by the dominant class. The history of medicine is littered with such examples. Cannabis, for example, can trace its medicinal roots to the "Himalayan region of central Asia[, from where it] spread gradually… to India, Asia Minor, North Africa, and across the desert to sub-Saharan Africa and the rest of the African continent" (Kalant 2001, p. 80). Whilst, given the lack of high quality evidence, I remain somewhat neutral regarding the effectiveness of cannabis's pharmaceutically active ingredients, early research suggests it is an effective treatment for nausea and vomiting and for the stimulation of appetite; that it is an effective analgesic, and potentially a useful anticonvulsant (Kalant 2001, p. 80). Cannabis also has significant cultural relevance for some communities, including the predominantly black Rastafarian community. But attitudes in the United States towards cannabis (exacerbated by Richard Nixon's "war on drugs"), arguably largely driven by racism (Montgomery 2023), prevented research into the plant's many medicinal uses for decades. Only now that the dominant social groups have begun to endorse it (it has become socially acceptable in many white communities, at least for medical use), is cannabis becoming legally available for medical use. It remains illegal in many of America's states, research into its positive health effects remains limited, and obtaining refined and reliably measured doses of the active ingredients remains difficult.

With examples like Cannabis, the route to decolonization might include the following: (1) incentivize medical research into both the benefits and risks of cannabis products, and if results are promising, develop appropriate affordable regulated treatments; (2) the harms *and benefits* of more traditional uses of cannabis (e.g. smoking) should be studied, and if deemed no more harmful than other legal drugs such as alcohol and tobacco, legalized in appropriate contexts, *bearing appropriate safety considerations in mind*; (3) the revenue from cannabis-related treatment should not benefit (only) multinational pharmaceutical companies, but also the marginalized groups historically targeted by anti-cannabis legislation.

However, a similar path is not open to indigenous interventions with no chemically active ingredients. Notwithstanding the fact that randomized controlled trials would be impossible for many of their interventions (pill bias), sangomas will not allow their practices to be subjected to western clinical trials. Furthermore, as previously noted, the evidential standards for TAM and western medicine are entirely incompatible. This leaves us in a quandary. Capacities-based principlism suggests that public health institutions promote the capacities necessary for the preservation of cultural heritage, and that includes (non-harmful) medical practices. It demands that the collective will of the population is respected, and given the popularity of TAM, it's fair to conclude that many African people want access to TAM. But it remains important that TAM be regulated to prevent harmful practices, and it's important to know what aspects of the paradigm are particularly effective, so its benefits can be maximized.

In response, I offer a tentative solution—albeit one that requires significant development beyond the scope of this chapter. I suggest that whilst the kind of clinical trials found in the upper echelons of the EBM hierarchy (such as RCTs) cannot be fairly applied to TAM, and the evidential standards of TAM clearly do not apply to western medicine, it may still be possible to evaluate the effectiveness of both traditions using another metric; one that focuses on the patients' experiences and capacities. One could apply something like Carel and Kidd's approach to good clinical practice in a follow-up context. Given that medicine is a patient-centric discipline, if the patient found value in their consultation, then the consultation had value. The assessment of their post-intervention health should be holistic. It should consider how they perceive changes in their capacities, both physical and mental (in other words, changes in their health, as understood in the book, should be evaluated from the perspective of the patient). It should consider the patients' overall experience of the consultation and treatment process. It should consider their perspective on developments in their "being". Studies could be done for a plurality of conditions, and those that offer positive results should be considered seriously by public health policymakers for public funding. Speculatively, I would be most optimistic about the potential for e.g. TAM to help indigenous people with mental health conditions such as depression and anxiety, through spiritual healing, ritual, and counselling. This being said, given the potential dangers, I do not believe public funding should be available for chemically active traditional cures that have not undergone appropriate clinical trials.

A similar approach can be taken to all public health interventions. Attempts to decolonize education, for example, should be closely monitored, primarily focusing on the student experience. Successful programmes should be replicated. Unsuccessful ones abandoned.

Like Harris's refined medical cosmopolitanism, the capacities-based approach to decolonization rejects medical relativism, and puts the values of patients and the cultures of societies at the centre of medical/public health decision-making. In addition, it suggests a new way of evaluating interventions from different epistemologies—one that is not prejudiced against indigenous knowledge systems. Of course, in the missionary example (where the missionary deceives the indigenous population into boiling their water through tales of evil spirits bubbling out), it's not clear that the capacities-based approach could do much better. Ultimately, the water needs to be boiled. It is an objective medical fact. However, the capacities-based approach nonetheless offers a path to a more inclusive and egalitarian healthcare system.

7.7 Conclusion

Attitudes towards traditional and western medicine among those who guide public health policy have far-reaching consequences. Thabo Mbeki, president of South Africa between 1999 and 2008, infamously questioned the link between HIV and AIDS, and went so far as to suggest that anti-retroviral drugs were poisonous. Mbeki believed that poverty (a direct result of western racism and capitalism) was the cause of AIDS, and concluded that this African problem required an African solution. As a result, South Africa was extremely slow to roll out the anti-retroviral therapy programme, and the country's life expectancy dropped from 62 in 1995 to 46 in 2002, largely due to untreated AIDS-related illnesses (Camp 2016). So, whilst there are plenty of reasons to decolonize public health, it should be done with caution.

That being said, it is undeniable that the harms of colonialism have persisted in postcolonial countries, and these harms will continue without active and intentional intervention. Decolonization is thus entirely necessary for a just society in postcolonial countries. The first step in this process is to identify the harms. The inequalities experienced by indigenous populations in postcolonial countries are often well-documented, and as I have shown, there is a growing body of literature on the epistemic harms indigenous populations endure, too. The second step, of course, is to rectify the inequalities and epistemic harms. In this chapter I have suggested that close adherence to capacities-based principlism will go some way to achieving this goal, so long as the perspectives of the marginalized are prioritized.

References

Adams, J. 2020. COVID-19: Blindsided by the pandemic experts saw coming. *Contemporary Sociology: A Journal of Reviews* 50 (4): 298–304.

Alkire, S., and J. Foster. 2011. Understandings and misunderstandings of multidimensional poverty measurement. *The Journal of Economic Inequality* 9:289–314.

Amiri, S. 2020. Unemployment associated with major depression disorder and depressive symptoms: A systematic review and meta-analysis. *International Journal of Occupational Safety and Ergonomics* 28 (4): 2080–2092.

Appiah, K. A. 2007. *Cosmopolitanism: Ethics in a world of strangers*. London: Penguin Random House.

Armstrong, D. M. 1973. *Belief, truth and knowledge*. London: Cambridge University Press.

Audet, C., et al. 2021. Throwing the bones to diagnose HIV: Views of rural South African traditional healers on undertaking HIV counselling and testing. *AIDS Care* 33 (10): 1316–1320.

Bach, P. B., et al. 1995. Variations in lung cancer risk among smokers. *Journal of the National Cancer Institute* 95 (6): 470–478.

Barnard, A. 2019. *Bushmen: Kalahari hunter-gatherers and their descendents*. Cambridge: Cambridge University Press.

Barongo-Muweke, N. 2016. *Decolonizing Education: Towards reconstructing a theory of citizenship education for postcolonial Africa*. s.l.: Springer Nature.

B. Smart, *The Philosophy of Public Health*,
https://doi.org/10.1007/978-3-031-98804-2_3

Bartram, J., K. Lewis, R. Lenton, and A. Wright. 2005. Focusing on improved water and sanitation for health. *Lancet* 365:810–812.

Beaglehole, R., and R. Horton. 2010. Global chronic diseases. *The Lancet* 376 (9753): 1619–1621.

Beauchamp, T., and J. Childress. 1994. *Principles of biomedical ethics*. Oxford: Oxford University Press.

Bedau, M. A. 2013. Weak emergence drives the science, epistemology, and metaphysics of synthetic biology. *Biological Theory* 8:334–345.

Beebee, L. 2011. A critique of hermaneutical injustice. *Proceedings of the Aristotelian Society* 111 (3): 479–486.

Berg, S. V., and d., Patel, L. & Bridgman, G. 2022. Food insecurity in South Africa: evidence from NIDS-CRAM wave 5. *Development Southern Africa* 39 (5): 722–737.

Berg, R. C., and E. Denison. 2012. Interventions to reduce the prevalence of female genital mutilation/cutting in African countries. *Campbell Systematic Reviews* 8 (1): 1–155.

Biggs, A., and L. Littlejohn. 2021. Revisiting the initial COVID-19 pandemic projections. *The Lancet* 2:e91–e92.

Bird, A. 2007. *Nature's metaphysics: Laws and properties*. Oxford: Oxford University Press.

Bloom, J. D., et al. 2021. Investigate the origins of Covid-19. *Science* 372 (6543): 694–694.

Boorse, C. 1977. Health as a theoretical concept. *Philosophy of Science* 44:542–573.

Boorse, C. 1997. Defining disease. In *What is Disease?* 1–135. New York: Humana Press.

Boorse, C. 2014. A second rebuttal on health. *Journal of Medicine and Philosophy* 39 (6): 683–724.

Branchflower, D. G., and A. J. Oswald. 2011. *International Happiness*. Cambridge: National Bureau of Economic Research.

Brennan, A. 2021. *Environmental ethics*. https://plato.stanford.edu/entries/ethics-environmental/

Broadbent, A. 2013. *Philosophy of epidemiology*. London and New York: Palgrave Macmillan.

Broadbent, A. 2019a. Health as a secondary property. *The British Journal for the Philosophy of Science* 70 (2): 609–627.

Broadbent, A. 2019b. *Philosophy of medicine*. Oxford: Oxford University Press.

Broadbent, A., H. Combrink, and B. T. H. Smart. 2020. Covid-19 in South Africa. *Global Epidemiology* 2:100034.

Brownson, R. C., J. E. Fielding, and C. M. Maylahn. 2009. Evidence based public-health: A fundamental concept for public health practice. *Annual Review of Public Health* 30:175–201.

Brownson, R. C., E. A. Baker, A. D. Deshpande, and K. N. Gillespie. 2018. *Evidence based public health*. 3rd ed. New York: Oxford University Press.

Brülde, B. 2011. Health, disease and the goal of public health. In *Public health ethics: Key concepts and issues in policy and practice*, 20–47. Cambridge: Cambridge University Press.

Buchanan, D. R. 2008. Autonomy, paternalism, and justice: Ethical priorities in public health. *American Journal of Public Health* 98 (1): 15–21.

Bulled, N., and M. Singer. 2020. In the shadow of HIV & TB: A commentary on the COVID epidemic in South Africa. *Global Public Health* 15 (8): 1231–1243.

Burger, C., R. Burger, and E. V. Doorslaer. 2022. The health impact of free access to antiretroviral therapy in South Africa. *Social Science and Medicine* 299:114832.

Byrne, E. Forthcoming. Epistemic injustice, medicine, and gender. In *The Oxford handbook for the philosophy of medicine*. Oxford: Oxford University Press.

Byrne, P., et al. 2022. Evaluating the association between low-density lipoprotein cholesterol reduction and relative and absolute effects of statin treatment: A systematic review and meta-analysis. *JAMA Internal Medicine* 182 (5): 474–481.

Camp, E. 2016. *Thabo Mbeki's AIDS denialism: Neoliberalism, government and civil society in South Africa*. lucas.leeds.ac.uk

Canguilhem, G. 1988. La santé: Concept vulgaire et question philosophique. *Cahiers du séminaire de philosophie* 8:119–133.

Carel, H., and I. J. Kidd. 2014. Epistemic injustice in healthcare: A philosophical analysis. *Medical Healthcare and Philosophy* 17:529–540.

Cartwright, N. 2012. Presidential address: Will this policy work for you? predicting effectiveness better: How philosophy helps. *Philosophy of Science* 79 (5): 973–989.

Cartwright, N. 2013. Knowing what we are talking about: Why evidence doesn't always travel. *Evidence and Policy* 9 (1): 97–112.

Caruso, P., et al. 2020. Diabetic foot problems during the COVID-19 pandemic in a tertiary care center: The emergency among the emergencies. *Diabetes Care* 43 (10): e120–e124.

CDC. 2022. Adult obesity facts. https://www.cdc.gov/obesity/data/adult.html. Accessed 1 Mar 2024.

Charters, E., and K. Heitman. 2021. How epidemics end. *Centaurus* 63 (1): 210–224.

Check, A. 2018. *Factsheet: wealth in South Africa.* https://africacheck.org/fact-checks/factsheets/factsheet-wealth-south-africa#:~:text=The%20bigger%20the%20gap%20between%20the%20mean%20and,average%20in%20the%2053%20countries%20studied%20was%202.5

Childress, J., et al. 2002. Public health ethics: Mapping the terrain. *The Journal of Law, Medicine & Ethics* 30 (2): 170–178.

Control, C. F. D. 2021. *Introduction to epidemiology.* https://archive.cdc.gov/#/details?url=https://www.cdc.gov/csels/dsepd/ss1978/lesson1/section11.html. Accessed 12 Feb 2024.

Cooper, R. 2002. Disease. *Studies in History and Philosophy of Science Part C: Biological and Biomedical Sciences* 33 (2): 263–282.

Dammann, O., and B. Smart. 2019. *Causation in population health informatics and data science.* s.l.:Springer: International Publishing.

Daniels, N. 2008. *Just Health: Meeting health needs fairly.* New York: Cambridge University Press.

Dignitas. 2024. *Who is dignitas.* http://www.dignitas.ch/?lang=en

Dotson, K. 2012. A cautionary tale on limiting epistemic oppression. *Frontiers: a Journal of Women Studies* 33 (1): 24–47.

Drewnowski, A. 2012. *The economics of food choice behavior: Why poverty and obesity are linked. Obesity treatment and prevention: New directions.* Vol. 73, 95–112. Karger Publishers.

Ellulu, M., et al. 2014. Epidemiology of obesity in developing countries: Challenges and prevention. *Global Epidemic Obesity* 2 (1): 1–6.

Epstein, R. M., and R. L. Street. 2011. The values and value of patient-centered care. *The Annals of Family Medicine* 9 (2): 100–103.

Fagerberg, H. 2023. What we argue about when we argue about disease. *Philosophy of Medicine* 4 (1): 1–20.

Fisher, D. N., and J. N. Pruitt. 2020. Insights from the study of complex systems for the ecology and evolution of animal populations. *Current Zoology* 66 (1): 1–14.

Freeman, S. 2023. *Original position.* https://plato.stanford.edu/entries/original-position/?trk=public_post_comment-text

Fricker, M. 2007. *Epistemic injustice: Power and the ethics of knowing.* Oxford: Oxford University Press.

Fuller, J. 2018. What are chronic diseases? *Synthese* 195:3197–3220.

Fuller, J. 2020. Medical nihilism by Jacob Stegenga: What is the right dose? *Studies in History and Philosophy of Biological and Biomedical Sciences* 81:101270.

Giroux, E. 2021. Can populations be healthy? perspectives from georges Canguilhem and geoffrey rose. *History and Philosophy of the Life Sciences* 43 (4): 111.

Goldman, A. I. 1967. A causal theory of knowing. *Journal of Philosophy* 64 (12): 357–372.

Goldman, A. I. 1975. Innate knowledge. In *Innate ideas.* Berkeley, CA: University of California Press.

Goldstein, B. D. 2001. The precautionary principle also applies to public health actions. *American Journal of Public Health* 91 (9): 1358–1361.

Gordon-Chipembere, N. 2011. *Representation and black womanhood: The legacy of Sarah Bartmaan.* New York: Palgrave Macmillan.

Government, SA. 2019. *Department of women on menstrual hygeine day.* https://www.gov.za/speeches/department-women-menstrual-hygiene-day-28-may-2019-0000#:~:text=In%20October%202018%20the%20Minister%20of%20Finance%20announced,1-3%20schools%20across%20the%20provinces%20of%20the%20country.

Griffiths, D. 2019. #FeesMustFall and the decolonised university in South Africa: Tensions and opportunities in a globalised world. *International Journal of Educational Research* 94:143–149.

Guerrero, J. D. 2010. On a naturalist theory of health: A critique. *Studies in History and Philosophy of Biological and Biomedical Sciences* 41:272–278.

Guyatt, G., and R. Drummond. 1993. *The users guide to the medical literature: A manual of evidence-based clinical practice.* Chicago: Americal Medical Association Press.

Harding, S. 1997. Is modern science and ethnoscience? rethinking epistemological assumptions. In *Science and technology in a developing worlds*, 37–64. Dordrecht: Springer.

Harris, C. 2021. "Science must fall" and the call for decolonization in South Africa. In *Global epistemologies and philosophies of science*, 106–114. s.l.:Routledge.

Harris, C. Forthcoming. Decolonizing medicine. In *The oxford handbook of philosophy of medicine*. Oxford: Oxford University Press.

Harrison, M., et al. 2010. The increasing cost of healthy food. *Australian and New Zealand Journal of Public Health* 34 (2): 179–186.

Hausman, D. 2015. *Valuing health: Well-being, freedom and suffering*. New York: Oxford University Press.

Headey, D., et al. 2020. Impacts of COVID-19 on childhood malnutrition and nutrition-related mortality. *The Lancet* 396 (10250): 519–521.

Health. 2008. *Closing the gap in a generation: Health equity through action on the social determinants of health*. Final report of the Commission on Social Determinants of Health, s.l.: World Health Organisation.

Hernan, M., and S. Taubman. 2008. Does obesity shorten life? The importance of well-defined interventions to answer causal questions. *International Journal of Obesity* 32 (3): S8–S14.

Ho, E. Y. 2006. Behold the power of Qi: The importance of Qi in the discourse of acupuncture. *Research on Language and Social Interaction* 39 (4): 411–440.

Hogan, A. B., et al. 2020. Potential impact of the COVID-19 pandemic on HIV, tuberculosis, and malaria in low-income and middle-income countries: A modelling study. *The Lancet Global Health* 8 (9): e1132–e1141.

Hume, D. 1739. *Abstract of a treatise of human nature. David hume: A treatise of human nature*. Oxford: Oxford University Press.

Hume, D. 1748 (2007). An enquiry concerning human understanding. Oxford: Oxford University Press.

ISS. 2020. *Instutute for Security Services*. https://issafrica.org/iss-today/police-abuses-during-lockdown-reflect-deep-accountability-problems. Accessed 12 Nov 2024.

Ivy, A. C. 1947. Nazi war crimes of a medical nature. *Federation Bulletin* 33 (5): 133–146.

Jazeera, A. 2023. *AlJazeera*. https://www.aljazeera.com/news/2023/5/22/in-south-africa-pupils-in-3000-schools-still-use-pit-toilets

Jenicek, M. 1997. Epidemiology, evidence-based medicine, and evidence-based public health. *Journal of Epidemiology* 7 (4): 187–197.

Jennings, B. 2007. Public health and civic republicanism. In *Ethics, prevention, and public health*, 30–58. Oxford: Oxford University Press.

Jiang, Dayang, X. Wang, and R. Zhao. 2022. Analysis on the economic recovery in the post-COVID-19 era: Evidence from China. *Frontiers in Public Health* 9:787190.

Kalant, H. 2001. Medicinal use of cannabis: History and current status. *Pain Research and Management* 6 (2): 80–91.

Kane, E. A., and T. E. Higham. 2015. Complex systems are more than the sum of their parts: Using integration to understand performance, biomechanics, and diversity. *Integrative and Comparative Biology* 55 (1): 146–165.

Karasek, R., and T. Theorell. 1990. *Healthy work: Stress, productivity, and the reconstruction of working life*. New York: Basic Books.

Kass, N. 2001. An ethics framework for public health. *American Journal of Public Health* 91 (11): 1777–1782.

Kerry, R., et al. 2012. Causation and evidence based practice: An ontological review. *Journal of Evaluation in Clinical Practice* 18 (5): 1006–1012.

Khabele, D., K. Holcomb, N. Connors, and L. Bradley. 2021. A perspective on James Marion Sims, MD, and antiblack racism in obstetrics and gynecology. *Journal of Minimally Invasive Gynecology* 28 (2): 153–155.

Khushf, G. 2013. A framework for understanding medical epistemologies. *Journal of Medicine and Philosophy* 38:461–486.

Kim, J. H., and A. R. Scialli. 2011. Thalidomide: The tragedy of birth defects and the effective treatment of disease. *Toxicology Sciences* 122 (1): 1–6.

Kingma, E. 2014. Naturalism about health and disease: Adding nuance for progress. *Journal of Medicine and Philosophy* 39:590–608.

Koch, R. 1884. The etiology of tuberculosis. *Mittheilungen aus dem Kaiserlichen Gesundheitsamte* 2:1–88.

Kolb, J. P., T. H. Oguin, A. Oberst, and J. Martinez. 2017. Programmed cell death and inflammation: Winter is coming. *Trends in Immunology* 38 (10): 705–718.

Kuna, A., and M. Gajewski. 2017. Cholera - the new strike of an old foe. *International Maritime Health* 68 (3): 163–167.

Ladyman, J., J. Lambert, and K. Wiesner. 2013. What is a complex system? *European Journal for Philosophy of Science* 3 (1): 33–67.

Lam, M., and R. Galvin. 2013. Effectiveness of acupuncture for nonspecific chronic low back pain. *Spine* 38 (24): 2124–2138.

Leclerc-Madlala, S. 2002. On the virgin cleansing myth: Gendered bodies, AIDS, and ethnomedicine. *African Journal of AIDS Research* 1:87–95.

Lee, Y. P., et al. 2020. Long term compensation of renal function after donor nephrectomy. *Korean Journal of Transplantation* 34 (2): 84–91.

Lemoine, M. 2013. Defining disease beyond conceptual analysis: An analysis of conceptual analysis in philosophy of medicine. *Theoretical Medicine and Bioethics* 34:309–325.

Leopold, A. 1949. *A sand county almanac*. Oxford: Oxford University Press.
Lewis, D. 1973. Causation. *The Journal of Philosophy* 70 (17): 556–567.
Liou, L., W. Joe, A. Kumar, and S. V. Subramanian. 2020. Inequalities in life expectancy: An analysis of 201 countries, 1950-2015. *Social Science and Medicine* 253:112964.
Ma'ayan, A. 2017. Complex systems biology. *Journal of the Royal Society Interface* 14 (20170391): 1–9.
Mackie, J. L. 1974. *The cement of the universe*. Oxford: Oxford University Press.
MacMahon, B., and T. F. Pugh. 1970. *Epidemiology; principles and methods*. Boston: Little.
Magness, P. W. 2021. *American institute for economic research*. https://www.aier.org/article/the-failure-of-imperial-college-modeling-is-far-worse-than-we-knew/
Marmot, M. 2010. *Fair society, healthy lives: The marmot review; strategic review of health inequalities in England post-2010*. Florence: Leo S. Olschki.
Marmot, M. 2023. Capabilities, human flourishing, and the weath gap. In *The Routledge handbook of the philosophy of public health*, 207–222. London and New York: Routledge.
Marmot, M. G., G. Rose, M. Shipley, and P. J. S. Hamilton. 1978. Employment grade and coronary heart disease in British civil servants. *Journal of Epidemiology and Community Health* 32 (4): 244–249.
Mercuri, M., and R. E. G. Upshur. 2023. Evidence based medicine and public health. In *The Routledge handbook of the philosophy of public health*, 143–160. London and New York: Routledge.
Metz, T. 2013. *Meaning in life*. Oxford: Oxford University Press.
Metz, T. 2021. Meaning and medicine: An underexplored bioethical value. *Ethik in der Medizin* 33:439–453.
MicrosoftNewsCentre. 2018. *Microsoft enables South African NPOs to drive greater impact through digital transformation*. https://news.microsoft.com/en-xm/2018/06/06/microsoft-enables-south-african-npos-to-drive-greater-impact-through-digital-transformation/
Mill, J. S. 1871. *Utilitarianism*. 7th ed. London: Longmans, Green, and Company.
Mohr, R. 1987. Aids, gays, and state coercion. *Bioethics* 1 (1): 35–50.
Montgomery, B. W. 2023. Cannabis policy in the 21st Century: Mandating an equitable future and shedding the racist past. *Clinical Therapeutics* 45 (6): 541–550.
Mothosola, W., P. C. Rathebe, and C. M. Mokoatle. 2019. *Stakeholders initiative in reducing mortality rates in traditional initiations schools in South Africa: A reflection paper*, 368–370. IEEE Xplore: Cape Town.

Mulder, R., et al. 2018. The limitations of using randomised controlled trials as a basis for developing treatment guidelines. *BMJ Ment Health* 21 (1): 4–6.
Mumford, S. 2004. *Laws in Nature*. s.l.: Routledge.
Mumford, S., and R. Anjum. 2011. *Getting Causes from Powers*. New York: Oxford University Press.
Munthe, C. 2008. The goals of public health: An integrated, multidimensional model. *Public Health Ethics* 1 (1): 39–52.
Ngubane, N. P., and B. Z. DeGama. 2024. The influence of culture on the cause, diagnosis and treatment of serious mental illness (ufufunyana): Perspectives of traditional health practitioners in the Harry Gwala District, KwaZulu-Natal. *Culture, Medicine, and Psychiatry* 48 (3): 634–654.
Nordenfelt, L. Y. 1987. *On the nature of health: An action-theoretic approach*. Dortrecht: Reidel.
Nordenfelt, L. 2018. Functions and health: Towards a praxis-oriented concept of health. *Biological Theory* 13:10–16.
Norway. 2021. *Scandinavia Stats: The Region in Numbers*. [Online] https://www.lifeinnorway.net/scandinavia-stats/#:~:text=As%20of%20late%20 2020%2C%20the%20population%20of%20Scandinavia,2%20in%20 Norway%20and%2025%2Fkm%202%20in%20Sweden
Nozick, R. 1981. *Philosophical explanations*. Cambridge: Harvard University Press.
Nuffield Council on Bioethics. 2007. *Public health: Ethical issues*. London: Nuffield Council on Bioethics.
Nussbaum, M. 2006. *Frontiers of justice: Disability, nationality, species membership*. Cambridge: The Belknap Press of Harvard University Press.
Nussbaum, M. 2011. *Creating Capabilities: The human development approach*. Cambridge: Harvard University Press.
Nutbeam, D. 2008. The evolving concept of health literacy. *Social Science and Medicine* 67 (12): 2072–2078.
Nyika, A. 2009. The ethics of improving African traditional medical practice: Scientific or African traditional research methods? *Acta Tropica* 112:S32–S36.
Ogbolu, Y., et al. 2022. Global learning for health equity: A literature review. *Annals of Global Health* 88 (1): 1–15.
Parfit, D. 1984. *Reasons and persons*. Oxford: Oxford Clarendon Press.
Peltzer, K. 2009. Utilization and practice of traditional/complementary/alternative medicine (TM/CAM) in South Africa. *African Journal of Traditional, Complementary, and Alternative Medicines* 6 (2): 175–185.

Phillips, B. et al. 2009. *Centre for evidence based medicine*. https://www.cebm.ox.ac.uk/resources/levels-of-evidence/oxford-centre-for-evidence-based-medicine-levels-of-evidence-march-2009

Pohlhaus, G. 2012. Relational knowing and epistemic injustice: Toward a theory of willful hermaneutical ignorance. *Hypatia* 27 (4): 715–735.

Porter, R. 2004. *Blood and guts: A short history of medicine*. s.l.: WW Norton and Company.

Posel, D., A. Oyenubi, and U. Kollamparambil. 2020. Job loss and mental health during the COVID-19 lockdown: Evidence from South Africa. *PLoS One* 16 (3): e0249352.

Ramsey, F. P. 1931. Knowledge. In *The foundations of mathematics and other essays*. New York: Harcourt Brace.

Rawls, J. 1971. *A theory of justice*. Cambridge, MA: Harvard University Press.

Rawls, J. 1993. *Political liberalism*. New York: Columbia University Press.

Rawls, J. 1999. *A theory of justice (Revised Edition)*. Cambridge, MA: Harvard University Press.

Rawls, J. 2001. In *Justice as fairness: A restatement*, ed. E. Kelly. Cambridge, MA: Harvard University Press.

Reading Panel 2030, RP. 2023. *Reading panel 2030*. https://www.readingpanel.co.za/

Reform. 2017. *Land audit report 2017*. https://www.gov.za/sites/default/files/gcis_document/201802/landauditreport13feb2018.pdf#:~:text=The%20Land%20Audit%20reveals%20that%20Whites%20own%2026%20663%20144

Requier, F. 2019. Bee colony health indicators: Synthesis and future directions. *CAB Reviews* 14 (56): 1–13.

Rhot-Arriaza, N. 1996. Of Seeds and shamans: The appropriation of the scientific and technical knowledge of indigenous and local communities. *Mitchigan Journal of International Law* 17:919–965.

Rivers, T. 1937. Viruses and Koch's postulates. *Journal of Bacteriology* 33 (1): 1–12.

Rocca, E., and R. L. Anjum. 2020. Causal evidence and dispositions in medicine and public health. *International Journal of Environmental Research and Public Health* 17 (6): 1813.

Ross, L. 2018. The doctrine of specific etiology. *Biology and Philosophy* 33 (37): 1–22.

Rothman, K. 2012. *Epidemiology: An introduction*. Oxford: Oxford University Press.

Sackett, D. L. 1979. Bias in analytic research. *Journal of Chronic Diseases* 32 (1-2): 51–63.
Sackett, D. L., and W. M. C. Rosenberg. 1995. On the need for evidence-based medicine. *Journal of Public Health* 17 (3): 330–334.
Sackett, D. L., et al. 1996. Evidence based medicine: What it is and what it isn't. *BMJ* 312 (7023): 71–72.
Samuel, O. M., and S. Mqomboti. 2017. Developing an integrative CSR model: Imperative for cultural and consultative dimensions. *Journal of African Business* 18 (1): 50–69.
Schroeder, A. 2013. Rethinking health: Healthy or healthier than? *The British Journal of the Philosophy of Science* 64:131–159.
Schulman, K., et al. 1999. The effect of race and sex of physicians recommendations for cardiac catheterization. *New England Journal of Medicine* 340:618–626.
Schwartz, P. 2007. Defining dysfunction: Natural selection, design, and drawing a line. *Philosophy of Science* 74 (3): 364–385.
Seeley, T. D., and P. K. Visscher. 2003. Choosing a home: How the scouts in a honey bee swarm perceive the completion of their group decision. *Behavioral Ecology and Sociobiology* 54 (5): 511–520.
Seidlelman, W. E. 1996. Nuremberg lamentation: For the forgotten victims of medical science. *British Medical Journal* 313:1463–1467.
Selgelid, M. J. 2016. Capabilities and incapabilities of the capabilities approach to health justice. *Bioethics* 30 (1): 25–33.
Sen, A. 1985. Well-being, agency and freedom: The dewey lectures 1984. *The Journal of Philosophy* 82 (4): 169–221.
Sen, A. 2009. *The idea of justice*. London: Penguin.
Singer, J. A. 2004. Narrative identity and meaning making across the adult lifespan: An introduction. *Journal of Personality* 72 (3): 437–460.
Singh, G. K., et al. 2017. social determinants of health in the united states: addressing major health inequality trends for the nation, 1935-2016. *International Journal of Maternal and Child Health and AIDS* 6 (2): 139–164.
Smart, B. T. 2014. On the classification of diseases. *Theoretical Medicine and Bioethics* 35:251–269.
Smart, B. 2016. *Concepts and causes in the philosophy of disease*. Basingstoke: Palgrave Macmillan.
Smart, B. 2017. Evidence based medicine and measurement. In *Measurement in medicine*, 3–21. London: Rowman and Littlefield.

Smart, B. 2023a. Concepts of health and disease in public health. In *The Routledge handbook of the philosophy of public health*, 53–69. London and New York: Routledge.

Smart, B. 2023b. Evidence based medicine and evidence based public health. In *The Routledge handbook of the philosophy of evidence*, ed. M. Lasonen-Aarnio and C. Littlejohn, 507–514. s.l: Routledge.

Smart, B., and H. Combrink. 2022. The ontology of epidemics. *Journal of Evaluation in Clinical Practice* 30 (5): 831–837.

Smart, B., H. Combrink, A. Broadbent, and P. Streicher. 2021. *Direct and indirect health effects of lockdown in South Africa*. Washington: The Centre for Global Development.

Sonnenberg, P., et al. 2004. HIV and pulmonary tuberculosis: The impact goes beyond those infect with HIV. *AIDS* 18 (4): 657–662.

Statistics. 2023. *Census 2021*. https://www.ons.gov.uk/peoplepopulationandcommunity/birthsdeathsandmarriages/deaths/bulletins/monthlymortalityanalysisenglandandwales/latest

StatsSA. 2021. *TB tops leading causes of death in SA in 2018*. https://www.statssa.gov.za/?p=14435

StatsSA. 2022. *Census 2022*. https://census.statssa.gov.za/#/

StatsSA. 2023. *Beyond unemployment - time-related underemployment in the SA labour market*. https://www.statssa.gov.za/?p=16312

Stegenga, J. 2018. *Medical nihilism*. Oxford: Oxford University Press.

Stevens, A. 2020. Governments cannot just 'follow the science' on COVID-19. *Nature Human Behavious* 4 (6): 560–560.

Stiegler, N., and J. P. Bouchard. 2020. South Africa: Challenges and successes of the COVID-19 lockdown. *Annales Médico-Psychologiques* 178 (7): 695–698.

Strotmann, H., and J. Volkert. 2018. Multidimensional poverty index and happiness. *Journal of Happiness Studies* 19:167–189.

Tate, A. J. M. 2019. Contributory injustice in psychiatry. *Journal of Medical Ethics* 45:97–100.

Temple, N. J. 2022. The origins of the obesity epidemic in the USA–lessons for today. *Nutrients* 14 (20): 4253.

The World Bank. 2022. *New World Bank report assesses sources of inequality in five countries in Southern Africa*. New World Bank Report Assesses Sources of Inequality in Five Countries in Southern Africa.

Thobejane, T. D. 2013. History of apartheid education and the problems of reconstruction in South Africa. *Sociology Study* 3 (1): 1–12.

Thomas, S. B., and S. C. Quinn. 2000. Light on the shadow of the syphilis study at tuskegee. *Health Promototion Practice* 1 (3): 234–237.

TimesLive. 2023. *TimesLive*. https://www.timeslive.co.za/news/south-africa/2023-05-26-newborn-babies-placed-in-boxes-at-hospital-north-west-health-mec-acts/

Tobi, A. 2023. Intra-group epistemic injustice. *Social Epistemology: A Journal of Knowledge, Culture and Policy* 37 (6): 798–809.

Toriola, A. T., S. Kurl, J. A. Laukkanen, and J. Kauhanen. 2009. Does binge drinking increase the risk of lung cancer: Results from the findrink study. *European Journal of Public Health* 19 (4): 389–393.

Valles, S. 2018. *Philosophy of population health: Philosophy for a new public health era*. New York: Routledge.

Varga, S. 2024. *Science, Medicine, and the Aims of Inquiry*. Cambridge University Press.

Venkantapuram, S. 2013. *Health justice: An argument from the capabilities approach*. Hoboken: Wiley.

Venkantapuram, S. 2016. On health justice. Some thoughts and responses to critics. *Bioethics* 30 (1): 49–55.

Wakefield, J. C. 1992. The concept of mental disorder: On the boundary between biological facts and social values. *American Psychologist* 47:373–388.

Werkhoven, S. 2019. A dispositional theory of health. *The British Journal of Philosophy of Science* 70:927–952.

Whiteside, A. 2002. Poverty and HIV/AIDS in Africa. *Third World Quarterly* 23 (2): 313–332.

WHO. 2024. *Constitution*. https://www.who.int/about/accountability/governance/constitution

WHO/UNICEF. 2020. *Joint monitoring report*. https://washdata.org/

Williams, T. N., et al. 2005. An immune basis for malaria protection by the sickle cell trait. *PLoS Medicine* 2 (5): e128.

Williamson, T. 2000. *Knowledge and its limits*. Oxford: Oxford University Press.

Wilson, P. W., W. P. Castelli, and W. B. Kannel. 1987. Coronary risk prediction in adults (the Framingham Heart Study). *The American Journal of Cardiology* 59 (14): G91–G94.

Wittgenstein, L. 2009. *Philosophical investigations*. Chichester: Blackwell Publishing Ltd.

Wolf, S. 2010. *Meaning in life and why it matters*. Princeton: Princeton University Press.

Woodward, A., and I. Kawachi. 2000. Why reduce health inequalities? *Journal of Epidemiology and Community Health* 54 (12): 923–929.

Index[1]

[1] Note: Page numbers followed by 'n' refer to notes.

B. Smart, *The Philosophy of Public Health*,
https://doi.org/10.1007/978-3-031-98804-2_3

Kolibri 360 GmbH
Ferdinand-Jühlke-Straße 7
99095 Erfurt, Deutschland
produktsicherheit@kolibri360.de